LEAVING DENTISTRY

A CAREER ALTERNATIVE GUIDE FOR THE
DOUBTFUL DENTIST

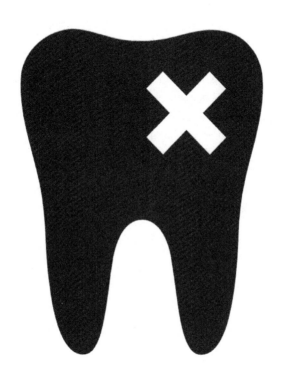

LEAVING **DENTISTRY**

Evan Blackwell DDS, Ms

Leaving **Dentistry**

A Career Alternative Guide for the Doubtful Dentist

Cover and Interior Design by:
Evan Blackwell

For my wonderful and supportive wife and son

Table of Contents

CONCLUSION   241

Introduction

Although no one can go back and make a brand new start,
anyone can start from now and make a brand new ending.

– Carl Bard

Young dentists entering the profession today feel as though they've been conned. I should know - I'm one of them. We were promised careers with four-day workweeks and complete autonomy. The men and women that we shadowed left school with practically no debt, opened a practice and enjoyed a healthy influx of new patients until they decided to retire. No stress, no mess, and clean teeth.

A dental professional today may not get the same impression of the dental industry. Instead, they are likely to see that millennials simply can't afford to open a private practice and work four days a week. Many dentists today have been forced to work longer hours, work under another dentist, or get bought out by a larger corporation. Dentists are professionals with years of schooling under their belts who must answer to micromanagers with non-dental backgrounds (or dentists who don't know how to run a successful business.)

A fifth or even sixth day at these corporate dental offices won't may not be enough when a dentist is shouldering $300,000 (or more) in student loan debt. Previous generations of dentists used to experience burnout within 20 years in the business. Now, dentists report burnout within one or two years.

Before entering dental school, I too shadowed professionals living in the "Golden Age of Dentistry." When I picked up my degree, I expected to quickly open a private practice, pay off my loans, and enjoy making a schedule with a satisfying work-life balance. These expectations turned out to be easier to envision than to realize. As an associate, I witnessed first-hand how the money that a private practice brings in can be *no match* for rising operating costs, heavy competition, and an overwhelming amount of debt. I turned to corporate dentistry but found additional problems there. The responsibilities of running a business were taken out of my hands and into the hands of someone with a business or marketing degree. Costs were cut, but often at the expense of the employees *or* the patients.

That's when I decided to walk away from clinical dentistry.

Even if you are not a dentist, you might still find yourself relating to these struggles. Medical professionals around the country are finding more work and fewer rewards in their chosen field. Teachers are experiencing similar rates of burnout. Millennials are replacing the "American Dream" with daydreams of working remotely, being their own boss, and working from a beach in Bali. A majority of Americans are dissatisfied with their current jobs. Some studies go as far as predicting that only 30% are engaged in the work that they are doing.

Unless you already work in a career that allows you to live as a "digital nomad," and work remote - transitioning is not easy. Dentists feel an immense pressure to stay in their field. Never mind the student loan debt knocking at their door - it can be anxiety-inducing and embarrassing to admit that you want to leave the field. If you were to broach the subject with your family, you might just get bombarded with judgment and questions. Why should anyone want to give up such a helpful and rewarding career? Why would you want to leave your private practice to work for someone else? How is going back to school going to benefit you when you're already drowning in student debt?

You might not have heard these questions out loud, but you've probably heard them in your head. These doubts haunted me as I considered pivoting my career. Without a community of dental professionals to support me, I wasn't sure I was making the right decision.

Any doubts I had about pivoting my career vanished when I became a father. My child has reminded me that life should not be consumed by work. A healthy work-life balance is necessary if you want to be present for your family, indulge in hobbies, and pursue your passions. I do not know many professionals in this new age of dentistry that feel comfortable with the balance that they have. Many have tipped the scales dangerously in one direction. Others do not know what balance is "right" and when it's time for a change.

How did we get here? Where is the working world heading? These are some of the questions that I'll address in this book. Recent generations have continued to invest more time and money into their jobs. As a result, young people are experiencing burnout way earlier than predicted. They have to make serious choices about how their career fits into their life. For some people, burnout is a sign to completely step away from a job and forge a new career path. For others, small adjustments can make the big difference they need to feel fulfilled in life.

What causes burnout? Why do we end up so frustrated with dentistry in the first place? I will begin this book by addressing the mental, physical, and financial toll that we put into our careers. "Time is money" is not just an old saying. Our time is valuable but is more often spent making up for the money that we have borrowed to get an education. Chapter 1 takes a closer look at the debt caused by student loans, and how changes in salary have not accounted for the changes in higher education. Debt puts a strain on the mental health of millions of Americans. Unfortunately, dentists and professionals are not stressed by debt alone. Chapter 2 addresses how high expectations, micromanagement, and isolation can cause chronic stress, which severely affects mental and physical health. Chapter 3 addresses the physical toll of the workweek. Hunching over patients for eight hours a day is enough to cause physical strains. But chronic stress can also exacerbate current physical conditions and increase the risk of heart disease, gastrointestinal problems, and obesity. Fortunately, there are ways to adjust your schedule and routine to counteract the mental and physical stress of a demanding job.

Why are we often required to bend our backs over patients for approximately *eight hours a day?* You might be surprised to learn that this "9 to 5" schedule was actually a relief for many Americans, although this weekly routine is often less fulfilling than promised. Why do we still abide by these rules? The answer is often entangled with tradition, convenience, and the rules set by corporate America.

Not everyone wants to follow these rules anymore. The chapter that follows reminds us that forging your career path is not all doom and gloom. We all feel the strain that a 40-hour workweek with increasing expectations has on employees throughout the country. Stress over debt, isolation, and doubts are not secrets. Chapter 5 shows the light at the end of the tunnel, partially illuminated by higher rates of remote work during the

COVID-19 pandemic. Although the pandemic has severely disrupted the routine of the working world, an increasing number of "digital nomads" and entrepreneurs have disrupted the 9-5 over the last 10-20 years. Now, these nomads have to take the world day by day, but their flexibility allows them to do so with limited levels of stress.

Ready to leave your career forever and forge into the unknown? Anyone in the dental industry knows that this is easier dreamed than done. Dentistry is not a career that people believe they can hop in and out of; dentists who want to leave often feel *trapped*. In this way, dentistry is like a cult. Chapter 6 breaks down why this comparison isn't so far-fetched, and how it may affect your feelings when it comes to leaving your career.

As you will learn throughout this book, the mindset of feeling trapped can be replaced with one that is more flexible. You *can* negotiate the schedule that you want and have the flexibility you need to maintain a healthy work-life balance. What does this work-life balance look like? This is the question we explore in Chapter 7.

A flexible schedule and a healthy work-life balance do not have to be unattainable goals. In the last three chapters of this book, I will address actionable steps that you can take to make decisions, set goals, and potentially make a career change out of clinical dentistry or direct-patient care. Not everyone reading this book will find that a new career is a solution for them. Instead, it might be more appropriate to look for a job with a different practice or re-negotiate your terms.

Whether you are hoping to re-negotiate your terms or step away completely, you must write out a solid plan first. Simply evaluating your salary needs, work-life balance, and passions could point you in the right direction. Will a salary increase eliminate the stress of student loans? Will a four-day week help you regain mental and physical health? There are many options to explore, a few of which are outlined in more detail in Chapter 9.

Ready to leave your job for good? Chapter 10 will show you how. Walking out the door tomorrow is not (usually) the solution. Saving, researching, and planning can help you immensely before you sign any paperwork. This book shows how much of an impact a job can have on a person's physical, mental, and emotional health. Hopping from one career to the next without research may put you in the same position this time next year. Proper planning is the key to finding a job that will bring you satisfaction.

Use this book as an opportunity to explore your current career and whether it fits into the life that you've envisioned for yourself. If you find that there is a disconnect, remember that you are not alone. Do not feel judged or ashamed, either. The increasing cost of education and the mounting expectations for associate dentists have prevented many Americans from meeting the expectations they have for themselves as a partner, parent, and person. There is an entire community of dentists, healthcare professionals, and other employees who feel the pressure of the 9-5. If you feel that it is time to leave, you have this community to empathize with and provide you support. Your life is your journey, and the path is not completely paved yet. *

*DISCLAIMER: The purpose of this book is not to bash dentistry nor is this book intended to persuade you to quit dentistry. If anything, this book is a guide to help you realize if leaving is even in the cards for you. Dentistry is a great profession for those who feel passionate about it. This book merely brings to light aspects of modern-day clinical dentistry that may not be palatable to those who do not love their career. I want this to be a resource and guide to setting career expectations and navigating negative feelings or matters that often arise out of feeling unfulfilled with dentistry. At the end of this book, you should be able to have a clear understanding about your personal and career goals. You should also be able to identify your passions and see if they align with the field of dentistry. If you find that they don't, this book will also assist you in motivating you to discover career alternatives that suit your passions. If you are just lazy or don't like working in general – then this book is not for you. Hard work, commitment, and purpose should be a prerequisite for any career, so it's important you understand that if you decide to leave dentistry. Moreover, working hard for a career you are not passionate about is self-abuse. The first step in ending this abuse is realizing and acknowledging the discontentment with dentistry that you hold and be able to share with others who feel the same.

Part I
The Burnout

Chapter 1:

The Investments Made

Most of you don't want success as much as you want to sleep.

— **Eric Thomas**

My colleagues and I believed that we had struck gold by choosing dentistry. The professionals that we shadowed were able to control their schedules, control their salaries, and enjoy working in an esteemed position. If we followed their same path, we would enjoy a flexible job, work-life balance, and a six-figure balance, too. Unfortunately, the Golden Age of Dentistry is over. Recent dental graduates have entered a field where everything appears to have dried up.

This disappointment hits especially hard when you've worked through so much to prepare for your career. Dental school is far from easy. Medical school is far from easy. College is far from easy, but a degree is required in most jobs that provide decent benefits and a hearty paycheck. Higher education is not just a place to open your mind and explore the world of academia. When you attend college, you are directly investing in your career and your life. And this investment isn't paying off as much as it did 20 or 30 years ago.

Unfortunately, more students find themselves asking if this investment is even worth it. Recent dental grads may not be "selling" the career as well as the dentists that my generation shadowed. After all, the point of an investment is to earn more than what you originally contributed. It takes years to earn a salary equivalent to what dental students take out in student loans. Paying off these loans in full requires decades of payments higher than the typical mortgage.

This chapter will go through the investments that young adults make today to pursue dentistry and other careers. The path between deciding that you want to pursue a career, and actually pursuing it, takes three things: time, money, and happiness.

Healthcare careers like dentistry require time. During this time, you are going to school, shadowing professionals, and studying for examinations that will allow you to enter the field or open up your own practice. The clock resets once you start working. Additional time is required to meet expectations set by the state dental board, attend continuing education courses, and learn skills that may not have been taught in schools.

Time is money, and the money involved in going to dental school quickly reaches six figures. Student loan debt has topped $1 trillion. Students around the country aren't just swimming in debt - they're drowning in it. Dentists face some of the highest student loan debts among any profession, forcing many to work longer hours just to stay afloat.

The stress of student loan debt comes with its own mental and emotional consequences. Working longer hours also comes with consequences. The idea of "eight hours work, eight hours recreation, eight hours rest" was coined in a very different era of American history.

An unhealthy work-life balance chips away at your happiness fast, creating a stressful cycle that ends in burnout.

As we cover these topics, I want you to remember that there is a way out of these cycles. This path may look different for you than for another person reading this book. But in order to understand your options and what paths you can take moving forward, it's important to evaluate what you have already invested, and what investments you may be required to make in the future. At the end of this chapter, I will provide exercises and suggestions for moving into a new life that allows you to enjoy more time, money, and happiness.

The Work We Put in Just to Work More

Wouldn't it be nice if you could walk into the job that you want and start working immediately? No advanced training, no special licensing, no changing your entire five-year or ten-year plan. You decide that you want a new career, and you go do it.

We all know that's not typically how things work. Even if you want the job you had when you were 14 or 15, you will probably have to go through an application process. A recruiter will look at your education, experience, certifications, the last place you worked, your background, your social media profiles, and your criminal history. Then, if they haven't already given the job to someone else, you can start to negotiate pay. If you are

13

new to the workforce or don't have many skills, that pay is not going to be high.

Landing your dream job takes time. If you are currently working in the dental field, you know just how much time it can take to legally practice dentistry or get a job working in a specialized field.

Spending Half Your Life in School

A career in dentistry requires almost a decade of your life before you can consider opening up a practice. You are lucky if this decade starts when you are 18 by registering for dental pre-requisite courses. If you completed an undergraduate degree outside the medical field, like me, it could take a bit longer until you can apply for dental school.

Dentists may complete dental school in four to eight years depending on if they specialize. During this time, you are studying for practicals, completing board examinations, taking part in internships, and considering whether you want to pursue more study in advanced dental education. This isn't just four years of school. Studying to be a dentist takes up every waking hour of your life at times. Even after dental school, there is required continuing education dentists need. (Sometimes, it takes up the hours you spend sleeping. There is a certain irony in a dental student having a dream that their teeth are falling out.)

The True Cost of Dental School

Requirements and standards to pass dental school have decreased, as well. One could look at this as a benefit, however in reality it is quite the disadvantage. The National Dental Board Examination has been changed to pass/fail, dental schools have gone from 50 crown and bridge requirements to 5 units, and some schools have abandoned procedural requirements and have gone to a portfolio-based system. As the required number of treatments is reduced for students, many graduating dentists do not feel like they have the training to confidently treat patients outside of the school clinic. This feeling can add to the weight of inadequacy and stress that new dentists bare.

This weight has become even heavier due to the overall reduction in the patient pool available in dental schools. Current dental students are struggling even to find patients to complete the requirements they need to show competency. Imagine paying hundreds of thousands of dollars to obtain a doctorate in a field you don't feel proficient in practicing. No wonder more and more young dentists are feeling discontentment with their situation.

Under Pressure

For many students, college is a time to let loose. Young adults are away from home for the first time and have the chance to explore the world around them. They're on their own, with a newfound freedom to pursue the life that they want to live. If you found yourself interested in dentistry, you not only have a specific plan for your life. You also likely have a specific set of personality traits. This includes the tendency to put pressure on yourself (and possibly the people around you): to be at the top of your class.

It takes a certain type of person to excel in (or even consider) dental school. Using the Myers-Briggs Type Indicator, *Dentistry Today* says that "ISTJs and ESTJs share many traits that make for great dentists. They're dedicated workers who value order, structure, and high standards. When they communicate, it's honest and direct, based on facts and logic rather than intuition and feelings." Future dentists typically have no problem with being detail-oriented. (Missing the small details result in big problems.) These traits matter because it directly influences how dental students prioritize and spend their time. They feel the pressure to continue their education *and* do exceptionally well. If you went to dental school, you probably weren't satisfied with simply waxing up a tooth. You wanted to be sure it looked anatomically perfect and that the occlusion was dead on.

This pressure, whether it is coming from yourself or outside sources, skews your priorities. During the four or more years that you are in dental school or residency, your number one priority is school. Everything else goes to the wayside. This is a hard habit to kick. Later in the chapter, I will discuss work-life balance. An unhealthy work-life balance rarely starts when you graduate or open your own practice. Many students have an unhealthy work-life balance that simply carries over into their careers. If you do not give yourself the ability to explore your passions or make time for hobbies as a young adult, it can be hard to make these parts of your life a priority after you graduate and enter "the real world." Career professionals may instead choose to spend all of their free time perfecting their craft, rather than exploring the world outside of it.

The Push Back

The "real world" comes with many milestones not related to your career. Once you have completed your undergraduate degree, other questions start to make their way to the dinner table and family parties. Are you having kids? Getting married? Buying a house?

Students in most degrees can approach these questions with ease. They graduate and enter the working world at 22. It's okay if they take a few years to meet their significant other and save up for a wedding, a house or kids.

When young adults spend extra time in school, they often feel a pressure to "catch up" and hit the milestones that their friends are hitting.

Sometimes these are milestones that your great-aunts and family friends expect you to reach and not ones of your own. The pressure to move fast doesn't guarantee a long-lasting or fulfilling relationship. Students feel torn. Do they take a step back to focus on having children soon? Or do they push forward with school and plan to start trying to conceive once they have a diploma? These are often the same young adults who are putting immense pressure on themselves to succeed. They want to have a perfect career and family - and focus on both at the same time.

Higher Education Means Larger Sacrifices

For many students, extra years of schooling wins out over moving forward with other milestones. Why? Time at school is an investment in their future *and* the next generation's future. The more time you spend at school, the more money you can make and put away in your child's college fund.

However, diploma might not feel like enough. Many dental students face a choice after graduation: stay in school for a few more years to obtain a specialty, or get into the workforce quickly. The dental field is no different. Do you want to specialize in oral surgery? Periodontics? Endodontics? If you are like me, there goes another three to four years of your life, dedicated to dental school. Yes, dentists can negotiate a higher salary and snag sought-after jobs with these extra credentials. But not for another few years (and thousands of dollars in loans.)

Ultimately, many students choose to enter the workforce. This choice does not always come from the student's desire to open their own practice or a lack of passion regarding a specialty in the dentistry world. "Choice" is often the improper term. The rising costs of education push people out of higher education and into the world of paying it back. Moreover, graduating dental students are starting their lives much later than their undergraduate counterparts, therefore there is an increased inclination to want to be in a hurry to begin living their lives after school; i.e. start a family, buy a house, go on vacations.

Dentistry Ain't Cheap

School has always been tough for dentists. The mouth has the same amount of teeth as it did 20 years ago. Less advanced technology was available to dentists of the past. Dentists of yesterday, however, had one less hurdle to jump: tuition. If you want to learn anything about teeth nowadays, you

18

have to shell out a lot of money. The rising costs of higher education aren't just a pain in the neck - they are pushing the country toward yet another financial crisis.

The field of dentistry also comes with the high costs of maintaining your licenses and practice. The costs of renewing your licenses, membership dues, CE courses, as well as paying for any new instrumentation and equipment you need for procedures. All these costs can start to add up, which is fine if you can write them off or your employer pays for them. However, there are many practicing employees and associates who have to foot the bill themselves in order to practice dentistry.

When Student Loan Debt Exceeds All Other Types of Debt

Let's turn back the clock to 1971. College tuition was already on the rise. If you wanted to go to a public school, you would probably have to shell out $8,730 for everything: tuition, room and board, and other fees. These costs were $10,000 higher if you wanted to choose an esteemed private university. Things stayed pretty stagnant until 1985 when the average cost for a public school increased to over $9,000. And then things started to skyrocket. By the same calculations, the average cost of public college in 2019 is $21,370. According to the College Board, private schools cost $48,510.

Look at dental school tuition over the last 50 years. The Journal of American Dental Association reported first-year dental student tuition costs incurred by state residents averaged to $3,311. Compare that with what the ADA currently reports for first year dental students at $37, 877. That is almost 10x the increase in tuition! At some point we have to ask ourselves are we getting 10x a return on this investment?

19

The rising costs of schools have led to more students taking out loans to pay for college. Seven out of ten college students today graduate with some form of debt. On average, that debt is around *$30,000*. 45 million Americans are currently trying to pay back $1.6 trillion worth of debt at an average interest rate of 5.8%. As a country, we owe more student loan debt than auto loan debt, credit card debt, and debt from home equity lines of credit. That's a lot of debt.

Has the country learned its lesson? No. Despite warnings from economic experts, the cost of college continues to rise. The College Board reported that private colleges increased costs by 3.4% between the 2018-2019 and 2019-2020 school years. COVID-19 has significantly impacted budgets for colleges across the country, forcing some to reduce their tuition and others to increase it at unprecedented rates. Even if a school is cutting tuition to bring back more students, it would take an ax to reduce costs back to what previous generations enjoyed upon entering school. Whether you strictly jumped into dental school or studied other fields for your undergraduate degree, you are likely to carry the burden of the rising costs of school.

The Dental Debt Dilemma

If you feel that you are drowning in student loan debt, you are clearly not alone. But I know what you're thinking. $30,000, the average amount of debt that students have at graduation, sounds like pocket change. You would probably love to have $30,000 left to pay. Student loan debt for dentists is much higher than the average student.

How much higher? Ten times higher.

According to data from the American Dental Education Association, the average dental student graduates with $292,169 of debt. Dental school students who attended public school owe an average of $261,305. If you attended private school, that average increases to $321,184. Almost four in ten dental students owe over $300,000, according to the American Dental Education Association.

■■

Dentists have to pay off up to $100,000 more than the average medical school student.

■■

If you want to compare dental school debt to other types of medical school debt, prepare to cringe.

- The average student leaves medical school with $196,520.

- If you went to pharmacy school, you're looking at something closer to $166,528.

- The average veterinary school debt sits in between the two at $183,014.

Today's dental students face an uphill battle after leaving school. While the average dentist's salary does provide some relief, it may not be enough to chip away at the mountain of debt that's accrued.

Debt Influences Your Job Choices

The American Dental Education Association offers some financing options and repayment plans, but they warn students to "never borrow more than you really need." I will also share some tips for paying back your loans at the end of this chapter and later in the book.

While there are options to relieve some of the weight, student loan debt is likely to put pressure on you for the next several years. The sheer amount of debt keeps many dentists in their position. Paying off $300,000 in 30 years at the average 5.8% interest rate would require a monthly payment of $1,760. In total, you would end up paying over $630,000. This plays a significant role in the jobs that you take, the salary that you can accept, and other big life choices. Student loans cost more month to month than a mortgage. No wonder half of all new graduates move back in with their parents.

Student loan debt also plays a significant role in how many patients we need to see and treat, which could lead to over-diagnosing individuals just to bring in more production. Dentists are spending more and more time at the office due to the increased need to see more patients and perform more treatment. Gone are the days of taking Fridays off. If you have ever considered adding a fifth, sixth, or seventh day of work to your week, you are not alone.

What You Can Do About Student Loan Debt

There will always be 24 hours in a day, and student loan debt will exist until it's paid off. There is no magic spell that will make your student loans disappear, but you can take small steps to improve your financial situation.

- **Assess your current situation.** In order to refinance your loan, you will need a good credit score and a low debt-to-income ratio. Get a feeling for where you are right now and what small steps you can make to improve your credit score.

- **Refinance your student loans.** Even if you *borrow* $300,000, high-interest rates force you to pay over $600,000 over 30 years. Refinance. Choose new loan terms and get interest rates as low as 2%. The higher your credit score, the more flexible lenders will be as you refinance.

- **Consider your loans in your budget.** If you do not have a strict budget right now, it's time to draw one up. Student loans will go away faster if you can pay off more today. Use apps like Clarity Money or Mint to understand how much you are spending each month and what expenses could go toward your debt.

Call your representatives. A phone call to Congress may not immediately reduce your outstanding student loan debt. But the call will be considered as politicians address the impending student loan crisis. If you believe that all loans should be forgiven, make your voice heard! Share your story with your representatives - yours might be the story that motivates them into taking action.

Finding a Work-Life Balance

No one gets a thrill from the idea of working five or six days a week. Dentists do it, not only to pay the bills but to meet rising demands from upper management or demanding patients.

Working outside of regular work hours often comes at
the expense of our happiness.

This is a cost that isn't always worth the joy that comes
from paying off your student loans faster. But what does work-
life balance actually look like, and why is it so important to your
happiness? This is what we'll explore throughout this section of
the chapter.

The 8/8/8 Rule

While "work-life balance" has made a comeback in
recent years, it is not a new concept. Robert Owen, a Welsh labor
rights activist who played a role in creating the 9 to 5, believed
that 8/8/8 was the perfect recipe for work-life balance. (You will
learn more about Owen in Chapter 5.) The 8/8/8 model
represented eight hours of work, eight hours of rest, and eight
hours of recreation. Unfortunately, these calculations do not fit
into today's society. Americans aren't just working more than
eight hours a day - they face responsibilities that take away from
eight hours of recreation and eight hours of work.

Travel, Traffic and Time Wasted

The commute to work alone can take away an hour from either recreation or rest. Americans commute an average of 26.1 minutes to work every day. These numbers vary wildly depending on your location and mode of transportation. In Austin, for example, the average commute is 40 minutes long. They rank third for the most stressful commutes in the country, following Miami and San Diego.

Austin and other metropolitan areas have other obstacles for dentists. When a dentist joins a practice, they have to sign a "non-compete clause." This clause forbids them from working at a practice within a specified number of miles; it may apply for *years* after a dentist leaves the practice. Dentists who are looking for other jobs may find themselves commuting farther and farther just to practice at a better job (or one with a higher salary.) Otherwise, they will face the choice of moving their entire life across the state.

Sitting in traffic puts stress on the mind and the body. You don't need me to tell you why traffic jams can cause people to yell and scream, but did you know that commuting can also increase blood pressure, and negatively affect posture? (I will go into the risks that come with poor posture and a physically demanding job in Chapter 5.) The longer the commute, the more health risks you face and the more time away from the things you love.

Speaking from personal experience, I was a traveling periodontist. I traveled to about nine different dental offices in the area that I rotated through each week. Luckily most of the offices were located about 15 minutes away from my home. However, I shudder to think if I had to drive to multiple offices, how much time I would have spent in the car. This is the reality for many people not just dentists. Even if you are unable to leave dentistry at this juncture in your life, finding a practice that is in close proximity of where you live will allow you to avoid wasting precious minutes in the car.

When the Office Closes

Dentists who stay within the state still have obligations to obtain continued education credits and certifications. Aside from commuting, the average professional dedicates time outside of work to advance their career. We have already discussed the many ways in which dentists maintain their licensure or continue their education. Unless you are employed by a corporation that will pay and give you time to continue your education, something's got to give.

Dentists who run their own practice may also face challenges outside of their patient-facing role. Marketing, growth, and paying the bills require hours of work (or hundreds of dollars to employees delegated to complete this work.) Some of this extra work is an investment into the practice, but some are simple maintenance. Rent must be paid, equipment must be ordered, and checkbooks must be balanced. If you are dedicating 40 hours each week to seeing patients, that work must be done outside of normal hours.

Making Time at Home

As any parent knows, "work" doesn't stop when you leave the office. Housework is still work. Data from the U.S. Bureau of Labor Statistics shows that Americans spend at least one hour a day on household activities. This number varies for men and women. Men spend one hour and 25 minutes each day on these activities, while women spend an average of two hours and 15 minutes.

26

Household activities include:

- Cooking
- Cleaning
- Laundry
- Household management
- Lawn and landscape management

The household chores don't go away just because you're exhausted from a full schedule of patients and treatment. In fact, often these chores can pile up.

Troubleshooting Time

Homeowners in recent years have realized that the time you spend on housework can be reduced without sacrificing a tidy space. How? Reducing the space of your home. The tiny house movement, along with other minimalist movements, has become a growing trend and response to calls for better work-life balance. Choosing to live in a smaller home can reduce the amount of time you spend cleaning. Decluttering offers the same effect.

At first, glance, adding minimalism to a book about the dental profession seems to be off-topic. But it isn't.

■■■

The solutions that you will find to your job satisfaction often lie outside HR policies or salary raises.

■■■

student loan debt, will not go away immediately as you decide to switch careers or obtain higher work-life satisfaction. Days will not exceed 24 hours. For every factor that you cannot change, there are multiple factors that you can change. Leaving dentistry may require getting creative. (I will be providing a handful of suggestions on how you can get creative later in the book.) Before you get creative, you have to re-prioritize and envision your ideal work-life balance.

What Does Work-Life Balance Look Like?

Dental professionals find it hard to adjust their work-life balance because scales tip differently for everyone. A single mother's work-life balance looks different than a guy in his 20s with no kids. Homeowners face different challenges than people living with their parents or young professionals sharing an apartment with four other people. Single people have different demands than people in relationships.

Regardless of your age, living situation, profession, or family size, work-life balance is about understanding where work fits into your life. If you are satisfied with how work fits into your life, you are more likely to be satisfied as a whole. When you spend more time at the office and less time with the "life" part of work-life balance, your quality of life is naturally going to dip.

Work-life balance isn't just a buzzword. Take it seriously. Although it's hard to define, work-life imbalances are easy to spot and feel.

■■■

Do you want to bring the stress of your job home, only to add extra stress onto your relationship or family?

■■■

28

Work can be stressful. Patients are draining, managers (or dental practice owners) are demanding, and there are physical costs to being on your feet all day. The more time you spend at work, the more time you spend in a stressed-out state of mind. Stress doesn't just "disappear" when you hang up your loupes and drive home. It remains in the body, wreaking havoc mentally and physically. I will go into more detail about the long-lasting effects of chronic stress in the next two chapters.

Your happiness and mood don't just affect you. It affects your partner, children, friends, and co-workers. This stress can then be recycled back into the clinic and affect how you treat patients and staff. Balance out the time that you spend at work and the time you spend enjoying your life.

Instead of bringing stress home with you, focus on ways that you can bring happiness from outside activities into the workplace. Calm, motivated energy is just as contagious as stress. Your work-life balance will help to lighten the mood at your office and positively affect your colleagues, employees, and patients. Work-life balance does more than help you. It helps your practice and the world at large.

Work-life balance is not so simple as dividing your time between work and home. Wikipedia's definition of work-life balance includes other responsibilities, including "health, pleasure, leisure, family, and spiritual development/meditation." We haven't even touched pleasure or leisure, much less meditation. As I mentioned at the beginning of this chapter, work-life balance looks different for everyone. In this final section, I want to talk about how you can envision a work-life balance that fits your financial situation, career aspirations, and lifestyle.

Take a Look at Your Priorities

When was the last time that you sat down and looked at your priorities? I am talking about literally sitting down and writing out your different priorities in life. You may be surprised to see that the areas where you invest the most time and money are not the things that bring you the most happiness. If you are not sure how to get started, try the activity below.

ACTIVITY: Circle all the priorities that you value.

Family	Nutrition	Personal growth
Friends	Fitness	Sports
Leisure	Success	Social media
Time	Fame	Meditation
Travel	New experiences	Humor
Dating	Music	Entrepreneurship
Education	Children	Mental health
Hobbies	Excitement	Marriage
Home/House	Self-Care	Career
Food	Religion	Pleasure
Spirituality	Volunteering	Finances

Which of these selections motivates you? Rank your top five priorities, and cross off anything that doesn't fit.

Are these the areas of your life where you are spending your time and money? Are these priorities able to be met with your current situation as a dental professional? Or are you letting other pressures and responsibilities get in the way?

Keep this list nearby as you assess the way you are living your life now and make a plan going forward. Put it in a place where you can remind yourself of what is important, even when things get stressful. Every priority requires sacrifice. When you remember *why* you are making these sacrifices, they will not become such a heavy burden.

In order to enjoy your most fulfilling life, you may want to make changes to how you spend your time and money. Don't start with big changes. Smaller changes can put you on the path toward a more fulfilling life. As I said earlier in the chapter, you just need a little creativity.

ACTIVITY: Take a look at your schedule. Where are you spending your time? How are you spending your time? Break it down hour by hour. Include any of these tasks on your list:

- At the office
- Notes
- Commute/Travel
- Meal prep
- Caring for others
- At the gym
- Grocery shopping

- Cleaning the house
- Arranging finances
- Checking your phone
- Sleeping
- Hobbies
- Talking to family and friends

TASKS	TIME SPENT
1.	
2.	
3.	
4.	
5.	
6.	
7.	

Record everything throughout the week. Check your screen time (found in the "Settings" on your phone.) You might be surprised to see how much time you spend in the car, scrolling through your phone, or doing household chores.

Once you record how you spend your time, you will likely see areas where you can *reclaim* your time. Set app limits on your phone. Delegate tasks to other people. Order curbside pickup for groceries to make your commute more productive. The possibilities are endless, and so are the possibilities of what you can do with this new time. Get creative.

How to Be More Efficient in the Dental Office

A lot of time-saving tips for the dental practice are focused on preparation and spending more time in the beginning so that you can waste less time in the end. Before you look at time-saving tips, it's important to track the current amount of time spent chairside and out of the operatory.

- **Digitalize Dentistry.** Utilization of an electronic health record (EHR) system like Dentrix or EagleSoft could potentially save a practice the most amount of time. You may think paper charting is a thing of the past, however, for many older offices it is extremely expensive to make the switch to digital or the owner may not want to learn a different way. Finding an office that has electronic records will be a sure way of cutting your in-office time down.

  If you are a practice owner, implementing a CRM (customer relationship management) program will allow for improved tracking and productivity from a business standpoint. Having the ability to track patient visits, treatment performed, automate billing, collection and budget reports could highlight ways to become more productive in the time given.

- **Morning Huddles.** Morning office meetings are a great way to highlight goals, potential issues, and solutions that may arise in the day. Discussing the schedule for the day also puts the entire staff on the same page, so that patient flow happens seamlessly, materials and equipment are ready and production is met. Without meeting prior, a dental clinic is prone to inorganization which leads to wasted time and potentially longer days.

- **Review patient charts.** Don't wait till the patient arrives in the dental chair before you look at the patient's chart or notes. Do they need new x-rays? Is the charting up to date? Do they need antibiotic prophylaxis or nitrous before treatment? Knowing the patient's history and needs before sitting down will save a lot of time rather than attempting to do it on-the-fly.

- **Sticky notes.** Teaching your assistants or staff to leave written messages is a great way to maximize efficiency when jumping from one operatory to another. This cuts down on having to locate staff and discuss who the next patient is or what the next treatment is and in which chair they are sitting.

- **Ready rooms.** Having all the equipment and instruments ready for a given treatment upon the patient's arrival will cut down on time wasted by assistants going back and forth to retrieve things last minute.

- **Scripted Talks.** Creating discussion guidelines or scripts for front staff and assistants will allow the team to communicate important topics to patients. Not only does this prevent staff members from explaining treatments on the fly and excessive talking but also potentially reduces the number of patient questions pre-operatively or postoperatively.

- **Calibrating staff.** Make an active effort to improve communication between front staff and assistants will prevent team members from running back and forth to collect patient information. This also ensures correct and accurate information is being described back and forth.

ACTIVITY: Now take a look at your work schedule. Write down a list of things that fill up a typical day in the clinic.

- Where are you spending your time in the office?

- How are you spending your time between patients?

- Are you mostly chair-side or spending all day writing notes?

DENTAL TASKS	TIME SPENT
1.	
2.	
3.	
4.	
5.	
6.	
7.	
8.	
9.	
10.	

Regaining Happiness

Take a moment to congratulate yourself for getting through this part of the book and taking small steps to enjoy a more fulfilling life. Doesn't it feel good to prioritize your happiness and regain control over how you spend your time and money? Keep these good feelings going. It's time to regain your happiness, too.

This starts with a simple mindset shift. Earlier in the chapter, I mentioned that certain personality traits are common among dentists. We seek perfection. We put pressure on ourselves to be the best and to provide. Although these expectations do not feel like a choice, they are. In the next chapter, I will discuss ways to step away from those expectations and regain a sense of acceptance for what is going on around you.

Anyone who has pursued higher education or worked overtime has already invested a lot in their careers. You deserve to make a return that exceeds what you have contributed thus far. If you are not getting what you want out of dentistry, it's time to pull out of this investment and focus on something that will bring you more time, money, and happiness.

Chapter 2:

Maintaining the Mental While in Dental

Working hard for something we don't care about is called stress: Working hard for something we love is called passion.
— **Simon Sinek**

D entists are not oblivious to the stereotypes placed on their profession. They know people are terrified of the dentist. They know that it's uncomfortable and ridiculous that they expect patients to have a chat with a bunch of instruments in their mouth. Patients say dentists "judge" them for their nonexistent flossing habits. While some of these stereotypes are harmless, one in particular troubles a lot of professionals throughout the industry. It's a stereotype known by patients, shared by healthcare professionals, and swept under the rug by dentists themselves.

People say that dentists have the highest suicide rate of any profession and if you're not a dentist, or you're entering the dental profession, this can be shocking. That's a pretty big claim to make and comes with some serious accusations about the stress related to the dental industry.

But dentists with a few years of work under their belts know that this isn't news. They hear this fact thrown around at cocktail parties, on airplanes, from strangers and colleagues alike. Suicide is not a laughing matter, but the supposed correlation between dentistry and suicide has been a running joke in the profession for decades.

Although there are no current, reliable statistics that show an increased rate of suicide in dentists, there are certain risk factors that contribute to the possibility. According to the CDC's list of top 30 occupations associated with propensity for increase suicide, healthcare workers (including dentists) come in at an 11.

The risk factors mentioned for work-related suicide include:

- Job-related isolation and demands

- Stressful work environments

- Work-home imbalance

- Financial pressures

All of which, dental providers can understand and have experienced.

Current data suggests that while dentists experience a high rate of depression and mood disorders, these may not lead to a higher rate of suicide compared to other professions. Even if dentists *did* consistently report a high rate of suicide, correlation does not equal causation. Careers do not solely influence someone's mental health or the risk of severe depression.

Other factors, including biological factors and stress from the world at large, can also contribute to depression. Even if you work outside of the healthcare field, you and your colleagues are not immune to mood disorders.

As we enter the new decade, many people have been forced to isolate and take on the mental toll of living through a global pandemic. Close to 40 million people lost their jobs. Others have lost family members, friends, and colleagues to COVID-19. Experts believe that based on the impact of unemployment throughout past recessions, 2020 could see a notable increase in the number of people who die from suicide.

Professionals across *all* industries should take the time to assess their mental health and how their employment status may contribute to the heaping pile of stress that is present in everyday life. A proper work-life balance keeps this stress in check. A *poor* work-life balance isn't just unhealthy; it's life-threatening.

Work-life balance is particularly important for dentists because the job comes with high-stress levels. If the stress of the outside world is carried into the office, dentists are more likely to make mistakes, lose focus, or become irritable. If work-related stress is carried out of the office and into the home, dentists will continue to be overwhelmed, frustrated, and subject to a cycle of stress and unhealthy behaviors.

In this chapter, I will address three sources of stress that are common in the dental industry. This includes the *stress to perform well* from management in corporate dentistry, patients, and the dentist themselves. A job well done isn't always reflected in one's paycheck: the loans required to complete dental school and open a practice eat away at a salary that has not increased much since the Great Recession.

Economic stress holds many dentists back as they plan for the future. The *stress of isolation and confinement* is not unique to COVID-19. Although dentists are not physically alone throughout the day, they are isolated from other people in their job position. Isolation and confinement, especially at work, can directly impact mental health.

At the end of this chapter, I will provide resources and suggestions for improving mental health in and out of the workplace. If you are struggling, do not be afraid to ask for help. It could save your life!

Perfection Stress

In Chapter 1, I discussed the specific personality traits found among dental students. They value order and high standards. Every detail must not only be addressed - it must be perfected. Dental school welcomes these high standards and raises the bar even higher, setting a precedent that follows dentists throughout their careers. The innate traits held by many dentists reinforce the pressure to perform well, and has them striving for perfection more times than not.

Striving for perfection may increase the quality of surgeries, exams, and other procedures. Unfortunately, no one professional is immune from the anguish that comes with perfectionism.

Changes in Perfection Stress

Although perfectionism has increased, perfectionism as a source of stress is not new to dentistry. In 1982, 1,000 dentists in the United States answered a survey about stress in dentistry. They listed the top causes of stress in the workplace.

ACTIVITY: Check the boxes to the left if you've dealt with any of them:

- Falling behind schedule ☐
- Striving for technical perfection ☐
- Causing pain or anxiety in patients ☐
- Canceled or late appointments ☐
- Lack of cooperation from patients in the chair ☐

These pressures were present even in "the Golden Age of Dentistry." This doesn't mean that one generation is less capable of handling stress than another. While the causes of stress mentioned above are still present, today's dentists experience more pressure and stress than ever before. Changes in the way that practices are run and how patients are managed make it harder for dentists to do their job successfully and satisfy everyone in the office.

New dentists face higher pressure and more sources of that pressure:

- Pressure to produce
- Social media reviews
- Pressure from patients
- Longer hours at the office
- Generational pressure

Picture this extra pressure as weight in a backpack. The race toward perfection, while a never-ending chase, is even harder to run with this extra weight.

Pressure from Management

Outside of the dental profession, pressure from owners or upper management feels like it's just "part of the job." Many aspire to "be their own boss" to alleviate that pressure and control more aspects of their career. This was a reality for most dentists in the "Golden Age of Dentistry." Stress from "higher-ups" was non-existent a few decades ago. Dentists never had bosses. After they graduated, they opened up a private practice and answered only to themselves.

Rising competition and costs of operating a solo private practice have encouraged more dentists to join a Dental Service Organizations (DSOs) or practice as an associate under an existing private provider. Dentists who choose this route are met with different challenges.

They Don't Teach You About Dentistry in Business School

Managers within DSOs typically do not have a dental background. Their degree is in business or marketing, rather than biology or dentistry. Their expertise is in cutting costs and raising their business's bottom line. Without the technical know-how, expectations and communication can be strained between management and dentists performing procedures. The choices that a dentist makes regarding a patient's health may not align with a business owner's desire to cut costs or overload the schedule. In addition, many dentists are now trying to balance

41

technical perfection with satisfying their employers. Achieving both is, at many times, impossible.

They Don't Teach You About Business in Dental School

When I left dental school, working as an associate appeared to be the best of both worlds. I did not have to shoulder many of the operating costs, but I would be working under someone who knew the ins and outs of dentistry. Associates still don't live the dream that many of us were promised at the beginning of dental school. Your success as an associate relies heavily on the owner of the practice. They may give you less flexibility or lower-paying patients and treatments. You may still end up taking on some of the operating responsibilities if you require certain materials or equipment.

■■■

Boundary-setting and clear communication are essential for associates working under a practice owner.

■■■

Pressure from Social Media

Dental school, despite its high costs, provides you with more than just a piece of paper. Patients or managers who do *not* have a dental education may get their knowledge from more accessible sources: specifically, social media.

"YouTube dentistry" gives people an "inside look" at different treatments and opportunities. Dental Instagram influencers, like anyone on social media, are strategic about what they post. They curate a feed that shows them performing advanced procedures (perfectly,) making tons of money and living the dream life. Notice that on many of these accounts, they only post their success cases and often without any mention of follow up or long-term results. If these accounts are your *only* exposure to dentistry besides going to the dentist yourself, you are going to have high expectations.

You have the ability to limit *your* social media usage and exposure to feeds that set unrealistic expectations for dentists. Unfortunately, you may not be able to do the same for patients, managers, or anyone else who may try to place these expectations on you.

Pressure from Online Reviews

Big dental chains handle operations and patient acquisition, giving dentists more time to focus on patient care. This shift takes autonomy out of the dentist's hands, but still ties the dentist's name to the treatment and patient's review of their experience. Patient reviews, especially ones written online, create additional hoops for any practitioner that relies on reputation or word of mouth.

Twenty years ago, online reviews were nonexistent. Patients simply heard about a local dentist through a friend and walked in the door. Dentists were more likely to be the only expert in their area, so the choice was even easier for patients. Patient acquisition and retention were not huge worries throughout the industry. Dental practices did not need to allocate a large budget for marketing, advertising, or public relations.

Competition has raised the standards and practices of dental offices in the past 20 years. So has the importance of social media reviews. Research from Moz.com reveals that a single bad review could drive away 22% of customers. Smaller practices with smaller marketing budgets are more likely to be impacted by bad reviews, although corporate dental practices will also see losses to their bottom line. Dentists are already striving for technical perfection. Now, they must offer perfect customer service, payment options, and timely service as well.

While most review sites allow the owners to defend themselves against negative reviews by commenting, you want to be careful about spending too much time arguing with "keyboard warriors."

Pressure from the Dental Board

When I tell colleagues and friends that I would love dentistry "if it weren't for the patients," I'm joking...for the most part. Patients control a dentist's fate in a way that doesn't always sit right. An angry patient could leave a bad social media review. If they're really fired up, they could file a dental malpractice lawsuit. Dentists also fear that patients take their frustrations to the state dental board. When these complaints are made, the board may step in with an investigation or even license revocation.

Why do patients leave bad reviews? Why do they make complaints to the board? Obviously, there may be legitimate concerns if a dentist truly screws up a surgery. But not all of these complaints should threaten a perfectly capable dentist's career. People get very emotional just *thinking* about dentists, and these emotions often fuel expectations, satisfaction, and complaints.

A survey from *DentaVox* lists the overall top complaints of dental practices.

1. Unexpected high costs of services and treatments
2. Quality of dental services and treatments
3. Long waiting times
4. Post-treatment complications and adverse reactions
5. Adverse incidents during treatments
6. Poor hygiene
7. Delays in diagnosis
8. Inappropriate behavior of dental staff
9. Use of old technology and methods
10. No or too little explanation about services and treatments
11. No or too little consideration of patient desires
12. No or too little consideration of patient symptoms

Note that many of these complaints are not even due to gross negligence, incompetence, or illegal activities e.g. drug use, insurance fraud, falsifying records. Even when attempting to do everything "by the book" a dentist can still receive a state board complaint and investigation. Many board complaints are from patients feeling dissatisfied with their experience not meeting their high expectations.
Some investigations even lead to record audits which could reveal non-germane concerns that require reprimanding.

High expectations from patients can be a major reason why some people become unhappy or irate after a dental visit. When you don't communicate thoroughly and set realistic expectations for treatment outcomes, patients could wind up thinking that their immediate dentures will fit perfectly and that it's your fault if it doesn't.

■■■

Establishing reasonable expectations also means effectively communicating procedures, alternatives, risks and answering any questions they have about their visit or treatment.

■■■

For instance, discussing potential post-operative discomfort a patient may experience after an extraction or reviewing the post-operative instructions, could save you from receiving emergency late-night calls from patients complaining.

Very few folks go to the dentist excited. People can develop a fear of dentists as a child and do not let go. (I have heard the phrase, "I hate the dentist" at least 1,000 times during my career.) This hate may give patients an unfair impression of any dentist they meet. Any and all uncomfortable experiences are placed on the dentist.

Sometimes, patients are upset with things outside of the dentist's control. Limited dental insurance forces patients to choose a practice, and this is often cited in complaints. One-star reviews may not even mention the dentist: patients are simply frustrated by the inability to schedule same-day appointments, the price of dental care compared to prices in other countries, rude receptionists, etc. Outside of the dental field, people are hard to please. Even if a dentist does their job perfectly, patients may still find a reason to be unsatisfied. One bad day or one mistake can stay on Yelp or Facebook for years.

Complaints to the board may be made years after a patient goes through treatment. A perfect job fails to guarantee that a patient will have a perfect smile for the rest of their life.

The process of striving for perfection does not end, especially in the dental field. Teeth do not "improve" over time. Even after a dentist perfectly installs implants or restores an entire mouth, maintenance of said work is out of their hands. It's up to patients to keep their teeth healthy and strong. A dentist's best efforts are no match for the natural wear and tear that teeth are subjected to throughout a patient's lifetime.

Dental Insurance Unchanged

If you are lucky enough to work for a fee-for-service practice then you can skip this next section. Let's review a brief history of dental insurance programs. Dental insurance was first established in the '60s with Delta Dental offering insurance at a $1,000 maximum in 1972. This could buy you an extensive amount of treatment during that time. Nowadays, believe it or not, the average max on dental plan coverage is still $1000 to $1,500. This means, that in the last 50 years, dental insurance benefits have not risen significantly to account for the increasing costs of dental treatments you recommend. This is insane if you compare it to other insurance models, like medical which has risen their cap over the decades. For whatever reasons dental insurance remains unchanged (which I won't go into in this book), it leaves patients and providers in a tough position when recommending and accepting dental treatment.

The truth is, dental insurance doesn't really operate as an insurance plan but more like a discount program. If the max coverage is $1000 on $5,000 worth of recommended treatment, then it's almost as if the patient is getting a 20% discount. This changes how willing patients are to accept treatment if they know they will be paying mostly out of pocket for procedures. It's hard as the provider to want the best for your patients but only be able to give them limited care due to their finances or weak insurance coverage. However, to reach more patients, we dentists have to sometime play by these rules of the game and be an "in-network" provider.

These programs not only affect how patients accept treatment but also how you the clinician diagnosis, prescribe and perform the treatment. Before insurance, dentists of the "golden age of dentistry" could perform dentistry without insurance dictating what procedures are covered. Now it has become a game of abusing the insurance policy to fit the dentist's needs at the cost of the patents. If you work for a corporate office or a private practice dentist as an associate, then you may have been convinced that their philosophy is the standard of care. However, it is important to understand that the production of the practice could be dependent on exploiting insurance codes to get the most revenue for their office. This type of practice makes good dentists do bad dentistry.

Malpractice Claims

Statistics have shown that the majority of dentists will be hit with a malpractice lawsuit at some point in their careers. Reports from the National Practitioner Data Bank reveal that among 19,755 dentists in the U.S., there were over 16,000 medical malpractice payments and almost 14,000 adverse actions filed against them. Moreover, these malpractice claims represent only those that were paid out. In reality, there are more likely a lot more claims filed against practicing dentists that resulted in no payout. It's important to understand the risks while being a dentist and to recognize the stress it could play if you decide to continue to practice.

Unpublished studies have also shown that when a dentist has a malpractice claim filed against them, that he or she is more than 5 times likely to be hit with another claim during the following year. It is suggested that the increased stress associated with being involved in litigation is what contributes to a second occurrence. As you traverse through your dental career, it's vital to have coping mechanisms in place to allow you to continue to remain focused and clear-headed in your personal and professional life.

MedPro Group has listed technical skills being a top risk factor in malpractice suits. This basically includes incidents of known treatment complications and poor procedural techniques.

Other risk factors listed for dental malpractice include:

- Behavior-related including patient dissatisfaction and non-compliance.

- Communication including patient rapport, managing expectations, and informed consent

- Administrative billing and collection issue

- Insignificant documentation of clinical findings or rationale for treatment and informed consent

If the possibility of being sued has been weighing over you and the decision to remain in clinical dentistry, you are not alone. Although the stakes can be much higher with performing dental procedures, almost all careers can be subject to litigation from the public. Finding ways to circumvent malpractice in dentistry will also help you develop thorough record-keeping and communication in the prevention of lawsuits in any career.

Medpro Group lists some helpful tips in avoiding dental malpractice claims:

- Try to only do treatments and procedures you feel confident in performing.

- If you don't feel confident in a procedure, you should write referrals to specialists to help reduce technical skill risks.

- Follow up with patients after procedures will allow you to better understand the patient's condition and tend to complications before arise.

- Document when you followed up with patients regarding concerns or complications. Comprehensive and accurate records of conversations and dates could be a lifesaver if ever involved in a malpractice claim.

- Diagnosis treatment appropriately by taking routine X-rays and periodontal probings to avoid having missed diagnoses. Recording specifics, like date, findings, and refusals of treatment, may be of benefit in any litigation proceedings.

- Be transparent, upfront, and set realistic expectations for your patients while explaining the treatment, risks, benefits, prognosis, healing/pain, treatment alternatives, and sequence of events.

- As communication among staff is cited as a big risk factor for dental claims, setting clear communication protocols will help resolve potential problems that could occur.

Although these are dental related, these guidelines can be boiled down to simple considerations for dealing with any customer or client in a career:

√ Have empathy
√ Practice timeliness to situations when they arise
√ Assessing the situation

√ Follow a response chain of command

√ De-escalate the situation

√ Understand when to act or when to seek support

√ Clear, honest, and open communication

√ Manage expectations

While these strategies may aid in avoiding malpractice lawsuits, these tips can't guarantee you won't be sued by a patient. Choosing to stay in clinical dentistry requires you to work with a trusted advisor to create an insurance policy that protects your assets, practice, and reputation on the likely chance that a lawsuit comes your way.

More Time at The Office

These sources of stress are more impactful as dentists spend more and more time at the office. Four days a week of stressful patients are easier to manage than six days a week of stressful patients. A healthy work-life balance mitigates the presence of these stressors in everyday life.

An unhealthy work-life balance also blurs the line between "work" and "life." When someone spends over 40 hours a week at their office, it's hard to brush off bad reviews. Attacks from disgruntled patients become personal, not just business.

It's no wonder that dentists and other professionals are experiencing burnout at high rates. The pressure to be perfect is exhausting. Without a proper weekend or evening to recover from that exhaustion, burnout is inevitable. Unfortunately, this is happening faster than ever. Dentists from the previous generation experienced burnout after two or three decades in the industry. Now, dental grads experience burnout within 5 years of practicing.

Generational Pressure

The pressure to be perfect is not just held among dentists or other healthcare professionals. Age also influences standards. Rates of perfectionism have risen sharply since the 1980s. Millennials face a higher pressure to be perfect, citing social media and the desire to earn a good salary as driving factors behind this pressure. Psychologists link these increasing rates of perfectionism to decreasing mental health. Chasing perfection is just that - a never-ending chase.

Younger dentists exiting schools are pushing themselves harder to complete that chase, and end up burning out within a few years of entering their field.

Hesitations About Seeking Help

This focus on perfection creates a dangerous cycle. Within that cycle is little room or encouragement to seek treatment. If someone was "perfect," why would they need to go see a therapist? Although treatment for mood disorder can reduce the risk of burnout, stigmas around mental illness continue to haunt people throughout all professions.

Later in this chapter, I will discuss ways to seek counseling that may be more comfortable than a typical therapist's office. If you are experiencing burnout, exhaustion, or anxiety surrounding your dentistry, you can benefit from various forms of treatment or making adjustments to your everyday life. Therapy should not be considered a "last resort." Not everyone who sees a therapist has to be diagnosed with a mood disorder or experience a mental breakdown. Seeing a therapist is not a sign that you need to be hospitalized or put on medication.

■■■

A monthly therapy session can simply help you put your career, priorities, and actions into perspective.

■■■

Do not let the stress of perfection get in the way of understanding and dealing with the other types of stress present in your job.

Financial Stress

Many healthcare professionals feel as though they are "damned if they do, damned if they don't." People experience higher rates of depression in a stressful job, but that stress does not go away if they lose their job. The true source of stress may not be the job itself, but the driving force behind going to work every day: money.

In the previous chapter, I provided data on the rising costs of college and what students invest in their future. The average student faces $30,000 in loans. The average dental student carries a burden ten times as heavy. It goes without saying that hundreds of dollars in debt can add an enormous amount of stress to every hour worked, every vacation planned, and every purchase made. Students enter careers like dentistry with the expectation that their salary will cover loan repayments. Unfortunately, dental incomes are failing to meet the rising costs of education.

Dental salaries hit a peak in 2005. The ADA reported that the average net income for general practitioners was $219,638. Student loan payments accounted for 16% of a dentist's monthly salary. Although the costs of college continued to rise, things looked okay for dentists entering the industry. As long as salaries continued to rise, debt and other costs could be manageable.

Then, the Great Recession happened. The average income for dentists dropped significantly around 2007. It has not come back since. In 2018, the average net income for a general dentist was $190,440. Since the Great Recession, dentists have experienced multiple years where salaries have remained stagnant.

Why Are Salaries Stagnant?

Shortly after the Great Recession, healthcare reform changed the way that dental care is provided. Dental care is not required under the Affordable Care Act. Patients must purchase insurance in addition to their overall healthcare. While the number of Americans with healthcare has increased since the passage of ACA, the number of Americans with dental insurance has decreased. As a result, fewer adults are seeking dental care.

Dentists are usually paid on production or collections. If they aren't performing treatments, they aren't able to collect any money. This system encourages dentists to stay open later and perform more and possibly unnecessary procedures. People may not seek dental care due to of their insurance, their fears, or a global pandemic. This leaves dentists scrambling to find and reach the patients that are available in the area.

Meanwhile, the supply of dentists is increasing, slowing the increase in wages even further. New dental schools are continuing to pop up and existing dental schools are increasing the number of available spots for enrollment. Dentists are also retiring later, giving new dentists with high loans less room to make a name for themselves in their local market.

One of the ways to combat the high supply and low demand in the market is to reduce costs. This directly impacts the dentists providing care to patients. In both private practices and DSOs, dentists are sacrificing their salary to meet rising costs and the slow influx of patients.

Fluctuating Finances

As most dentists are paid on production from the previous month, it's not uncommon to have each paycheck be different from the next. A good month of seeing patients and performing treatments could potentially mean double income that month. However, due to unforeseen circumstances (like a global pandemic), a slow office could mean half the production which results in half your income. The variability of amounts being paid could lead to challenges in adequately budgeting or saving while trying to pay off student loans. Consider if finding a career that has a more fixed salary dispersed each pay period would be better for your long-term economic happiness.

Paying Off Loans Today

Stagnant salaries pose a challenge for graduates who are paying back loans with 5.8% interest. A monthly $3,000 payment eats up over 18% of the average dentist's monthly income. This can be discouraging, especially when a typical budget breakdown doesn't account for debt repayment. (The typical 50/30/20 breakdown leaves 20% of one's monthly salary for debt repayment *and* savings.) No wonder dentists are trying to squeeze in extra hours and make extra money. It often feels as if there is no other choice.

Income-based repayment (IBR) plans are an option for dentists whose payments exceed 20% of their monthly income. Unfortunately, they come at a price. Income-driven repayment plans may reduce your monthly payment to 10% or 20%. Your loans will be forgiven - but only if you make consistent payments over 20 to 25 years. Not all dentists will benefit from income-driven repayment plans, but it might be worth considering.

The StudentLoanPlanner.com reports there are the two best ways for dentist professionals to eliminate or reduce student loans:

1. **Aggressive Pay Back.** For dentists who owe 1.5 times their income or less, it's recommended that they put every penny they can afford at paying down on their debt until it is paid.

2. **Pay the least amount possible.** For dentists who owe more than twice their income, the goal is to apply for an income-driven repayment plan that will maintain low payments and take advantage of taxable loan forgiveness.

Which option is best will depend on where your office is located and if you own it or not. Consolidating loans and refinancing to get a lower rate also provides an opportunity to pay off loans faster without as much interest.

After researching long and hard about what paying off student loan debt for me looked like after finishing residency, I determined the best option was 2. This led me to choose the income-based repayment plan called "Pay As You Earn" or PAYE.

StudentLoanPlanner.com lists some of the pros and cons of PAYE and refinancing to help guide you on managing your student loan debt:

PAYE

- **Pro:** Affordable monthly payments, which will allow you to save, invest, and put money toward other financial goals.
- **Pro:** 20 years to save up for taxes owed.
- **Con:** His loan balance will grow from $300,000 to $433,000.
- **Con:** May take longer to pay off compared to refinancing.

REFINANCING

- **Pro:** Possibility of being out of debt faster.
- **Pro:** Possibility of paying less in total loans.
- **Con:** Once you refinance, federal loan program benefits, like IBR plans, are gone for good.
- **Con:** You could be stuck with a high monthly loan payment without the flexibility to change.

PAYE was able to provide me with the flexibility and lower payments to achieve the financial goals I had, i.e. starting a family, and buying a home. However, I am fully aware that my loan will continue to grow for the next 20 years until being eligible for taxable forgiveness.

Other Ways to Handle Economic Stress

The stress of student loans and a stagnant salary can be overwhelming, but it should not be ignored. Money is a significant source of stress for all Americans. Psychologists suggest that it could be more stressful than the average workday or relationships at home. Your mental and physical health may not get better if you do not tackle the sources of chronic stress.

Overcoming financial stress requires facing it. I will continue to provide suggestions on repaying debt, negotiating for a higher salary, and budgeting throughout this book. Everyone's financial situation is different, forcing everyone to take different paths toward no debt and consistent cash flow. No matter what your financial situation looks like, it's time to take action.

Creating a budget with the use of software like *Mint.com* is an easy way to track and manage your personal finances in order to successfully pay down your dental student loan debt.

Isolation and Confinement

Sources of stress attributed to isolation or confinement became even more exaggerated in the early months of 2020. When COVID-19 sent millions of Americans into isolation, experts at the Centers for Disease Control warned that there was more at risk than contracting a virus. The CDC states social isolation and loneliness are high-risk factors in depression and suicide.

Unfortunately, these feelings of isolation are not new for dentists. Even in the "Golden Age of Dentistry," dentists cited isolation as a source of stress. Professionals who "work alone" often find themselves experiencing the symptoms of isolation.

Why Do Dentists Feel So Isolated?

A dentist's office may be buzzing with people all day long, but that does not shield dentists, hygienists, or any other staff from experiencing loneliness. As I mentioned earlier in the chapter, patients do not always bring warm and fuzzy feelings with them. After you've heard, "I hate the dentist," for the 1,000th time, you start to believe that *everyone* who walks into the office has similar feelings. It eventually starts to wear on your morale. We know that small talk does not fully help patients overcome this fear, as they are unable to talk with the tools and hands in their mouth. The relationship that dentists have with their patients is very different from say, salesmen, and regular customers.

There is little time for pleasantries or social conversation, especially when dentists are trying to fit in more patients. This doesn't mean that dentists are unable to build rapport with their patients, it just means it has become more challenging with modern-day dental pressures. Between patients, dentists retreat to their office to write notes, look at charts, and manage the operations of their business. In the office, dentists are typically alone as the sole provider.

They have little time to vent (or share good stories) of patients or their day. Dentists feel pressure to perform perfectly from patients, managers, and society at large. Sharing their own personal fears, or reaching out with questions, feels like an admittance of failure. The only other dentists you may see all day are the "perfect" ones on social media. They're going to be the last people to admit, to tens of thousands of followers, that they aren't happy or feel like they could do better. High expectations put the pressure and the blame on the individual dentists. If something "goes wrong," dentists fear that others will see them as lazy, weak, or uneducated. No one is perfect, but there appears to be very little room for imperfection in the world of dentistry.

When dentists spend more hours on the job, these feelings of isolation and loneliness take up more and more of their day.

The Dangers of Isolation

If someone is feeling lonely at work but has to spend more and more time in the office, loneliness becomes a prominent feeling in that person's life. Loneliness isn't just a nagging sadness - it poses dangerous risks.

In fact, public health experts are calling loneliness an "epidemic." Studies show that social isolation and loneliness can increase premature mortality and the risk of conditions like cardiovascular disease, dementia, depression, and anxiety. In recent years, the risks of loneliness have been equated to smoking 15 cigarettes a day. Experts believe that loneliness is just as dangerous as obesity and inactivity.

Other Factors That Contribute to Loneliness

I mentioned at the beginning of this chapter that employment status is far from the only factor contributing to mental illness. Pressure and isolation due to work certainly serve as a large source of stress, but employees must take a look outside work to understand their feelings, too. Loneliness is not a feeling that is reserved for the office, especially amongst young people.

Social media, for example, has been tied to the "loneliness epidemic." Although social media platforms give those the opportunity to reach new people, it is often used as a substitute for in-person interaction. The images that we see on social media often reflect an inflated lifestyle. Seeing friends and colleagues in their best moments make many social media users question where they stand. Filtered selfies and vacation photos make it hard to compare ourselves to others - and come out on top.

Regardless of your job position, salary, number of followers on Instagram, or student loan debt, loneliness may creep into your mind and impact your mental health.

■■

It's time to assess your mental health, how it is impacted by your lifestyle, and the ways to alleviate pressure and other sources of chronic stress.

■■

It may be time to delete some of these influencer accounts or at least assess them to see if the content they are displaying adds positivity to your feed. If not, then try you'll need to make an active effort to follow more accounts or groups that allow you to feel connected but don't leave you envious or competitive.

How to Handle Stress of Expectations, Economics, and Isolation

Chronic stress is not just an issue of mental health. Physical health is directly influenced by mental health. An overwhelming job can disrupt sleep patterns, encourage physical inactivity, or increase the risk of other harmful habits. From afar, it's easy to connect the high rates of stress in the dental industry to serious health conditions. Suicide rates are not the number one killer of dentists, but this doesn't mean mental health is not severely impacting professionals in the industry. The number one killer of dentists is stress-related cardiovascular disease.

If you are experiencing high levels of stress at work, take action. Consider it as an effort to improve your physical, mental, and emotional health. In the long run, reducing chronic stress will greatly benefit these different areas and your overall wellbeing. Before we discuss ways we can prevent or reduce stress it's important to recognize what areas of dentistry stress us out.

ACTIVITY: Rank the levels of stress affecting you that are commonly associated with dentistry.

_____ Time/Schedule Pressures
_____ Patient Demands and Disappointment
_____ Uncooperative or Anxious Patients
_____ High Levels of Concentration or Focus
_____ Fear of Malpractice Suit
_____ Fear of State Board Complaints
_____ Team and Staff Issues
_____ Pressure to perform quality treatment
_____ Making production goals
_____ Isolation
_____ Student Loan Debt

Coping with the Stress

Even though stress feels like one overwhelming emotion, it comes from many sources. High expectations, economic burdens, and a lack of social interaction all contribute to a cycle of comparison, disappointment, and stress. This cycle, however, can be broken. The first step to managing chronic stress is to believe that this can be accomplished.

Do not let these statistics paint a hopeless picture of chronic stress and mental health. None of the contributing factors mentioned in this chapter are biological. They are not set in stone. It is possible to take certain actions (even small ones) to remove yourself from this cycle and enjoy a more fulfilling and optimistic life.

Not everyone has to pursue mental health counseling or therapy in order to relieve stress. Time and money management may be the keys to alleviating the pressures of the workplace and reducing your risk of stress-related conditions.

TIPS:

- **Track your stressors.** Start writing down in a journal times where you felt most stress and how you dealt with them. Document your thoughts, feelings, and any information about the situation. Tracking things can help you find commonalities between your stressors and how you react to them.

- **Develop healthy responses.** Don't fight stress and anxiety with unhealthy food or alcohol. Try to make healthy choices when demanding situations come up. Exercise is a great way to cut stress. Also make time for hobbies and favorite activities, like reading or playing games. Building healthy habits like getting enough good-quality sleep and reducing stimulating TV or computer usage are important for successful stress management.

- **Establish boundaries.** Create work-life boundaries for yourself. It's okay if you don't check your email at home in the evening, or if you don't answer the phone while eating dinner. Establishing clear boundaries work and home can reduce the potential for conflict between the two and the stress arises because of it.

- **Take time to recharge.** Stress and burnout usually occur when we haven't had a break. Once you disconnect from the clinic every once and a while, you'll find that by taking time off to relax and unwind, you return to work revitalized and productive.

- **Learn how to relax.** Meditation, deep breathing exercises, and mindfulness are proven ways to take control to become calm and aware of your stressors. The ability to focus on one activity without distraction will not only decrease your anxiety but also benefit other aspects of your life.

- **Talk to your supervisor.** Employee health has been linked to productivity at work, so your boss has an incentive to create a work environment that promotes employee well-being. Have a conversation with your manager or the practice owner to develop with a strategy for dealing with the stressors you've identified, which will help you be a productive employee.

- **Get some support.** Get support from trustworthy friends and family. They may have helpful ways to manage stress. Check with your employer or HR for resources on stress management, if needed. Lastly, seeking professional assistance with managing stress can be obtained by talking to a licensed counselor or therapist who can lessen unhealthy behavior associated with stress.

How Much Time Do You Spend on Hobbies?

In previous decades, golf was a popular hobby among dentists. This pastime allowed dentists to stay active, connect with other dentists, and let off some steam. Dentistry is a stressful profession whether you are working three, four, or six days a week. Hobbies like golf allow dentists to relieve stress and have a healthy work-life balance. Nowadays, dentists feel pressured to skip the sport and spend more time operating on patients, researching new dental techniques or implementing practice management protocols.

If you are experiencing an unhealthy work-life balance, you are more likely to spend your time in the office and less time socializing, enjoying leisure, and pursuing outside passions. As you make room in your schedule for time outside of work, leave some room to pursue a hobby or passion. You don't have to play golf. Find *some* way to reduce always thinking about dentistry and spend more time pursuing a passion or hobby that steers you to happiness.

When I say "hobby," I'm not talking about a side hustle. Hobbies do not make a profit. Find an activity that purely brings you joy. Not sure where to start? Explore! High demands from higher education often put this phase of exploration on the back burner.

■■■I

If you don't have a hobby, enjoy the process of trying new things, having new experiences, and relieving some stress along the way.

■■■I

Do not worry about your skill level or how this hobby can pay off in the future. You do not have to be a perfect golfer to plan a monthly game with friends. You don't need to have the fanciest bike or go on cross-country trips to enjoy cycling. Choose something that makes the time go by fast and gives you an escape from the pressures of work. Remember, both active *and* non-active hobbies can benefit your mental (and therefore physical) health. Quilting, breadmaking, and reading can all help you unwind and recover from stress.

You might say, "Between work and having a family, I don't have any time!" While it's true that having children to raise or other priorities can require a substantial portion of your time, there are always ways to increase the amount of hours in your day.

1. **Wake Up Earlier.** If you are used to waking up at 8 am, think about how much more productive you could be at 5:30 am.

2. **Prepare.** The more organized you are, the more efficient you can be in your day. This includes writing a to-do list or meal prepping for the week.

3. **Delegate.** Assign tasks or split responsibilities with co-workers or family members.

4. **Utilize Tools.** Downloading apps that help automate areas of your life will greatly increase time throughout the day. Find apps that sync your calendar with daily tasks or your notes. Apps that prepare your exercise routine or nutrition for the day will prevent wasted time thinking about it. There are even apps that analyze how much time you spend on your phone.

5. **Discover Time Suckers.** Find out what moments in your day are spent excessively watching TV or on social media. What may seem like a small amount of time, once you quantify it – you may see you spend more than you think.

Reducing Stress and Expectations at Work

With a clear mind and fresh eyes, you can go into work and find ways to relieve stress in the office. Take some time to analyze how you spend your time *in* the office. How many patients are you seeing? How many procedures are you trying to squeeze into one day? If you're not a dentist yet, at what point do you find yourself overwhelmed by the amount of tasks piled up on your desk?

Pinpoint what is stressing you out, and when this stress starts to affect your work. This will look different for every professional. Your limit may look different from other people in your field or your office and that is okay.

Once you have identified your breaking points, set boundaries, and expectations. Regain control over your day. Saying "no," reducing your load, or referring patients out to other professionals is not going to be easy. But remember the bigger picture. When you spend less time at work stressed over your workload, you set yourself up for a healthier work-life balance.

Boundary-setting is a practice that will benefit you *outside* the workplace.

■■

Control your schedule at work and you can have more control over your schedule in life.

■■

Take It Easy

Reducing your workload can play a significant role in preventing burnout, but it will not make all of your worries go away. If you still feel overwhelmed at work or home, you have many options for treatment and managing your emotions in a healthy manner, like counseling, yoga or meditation.

Career Counseling

Tackle specific work-related stress with a career coach or counselor. These coaches do more than help you look for a new job. They often provide negotiation advice, interview tips, and insight into specific careers. A session with a career coach may help you remember *why* you chose your job, or help you make the decision to actually leave dentistry.

Practice Management Consulting

There are a multitude of dental practice management programs out there to help you achieve your practice goals while staying in clinical dentistry. These programs are geared to increase revenue while decreasing the number of patients you see. If this is only what it takes for you to be happy with dentistry then finding a trusted practice management consultant may be the key. However, buyer beware. I know many dentists who have spent thousands of dollars on these programs that offer many promises and don't quite deliver.

Professional Therapy

Speaking to an objective, third-party professional can help you sort through issues at work and at home in a confidential manner. Therapy is not a sign of weakness; rather, it's a step toward a healthier relationship with yourself, your family, and your work.

Therapists are not all the same. Each therapist may take a different approach to mental health counseling. While some therapists may specialize in work-related conflicts, others specialize in family counseling. You can also find therapists that specialize in anxiety, LGBTQ issues, trauma counseling, or recovering from disordered eating.

In the wake of COVID-19, more therapists are taking their practice online. Talk therapy is available through individual practices or larger companies like *BetterHealth*. Speak to a therapist on your own time, as often as you need. Some insurance companies even cover mental health counseling. Typically, copayments count toward your deductible or out-of-pocket maximum. Check with your insurance company before reaching out to a local therapist.

Meditation

Therapists will suggest tools and exercises that will help you manage stress outside of the therapist's office. One of these practices is meditation. A few minutes of meditation each day can help you refocus, boost your mood, or manage stress in your body and mind.

Some dental schools like Oregon Health and Sciences University have installed 'Meditation Rooms.' These are areas built in newer dental schools that are a quiet space with mats and pillows where dental students can take a minute to breathe and relax.

Meditation is not just sitting in a room chanting or "thinking of nothing." Teachers often remind students that thoughts and worries come and go. You can still "successfully" meditate, even if your brain is full of chatter and you're sitting in an office surrounded by the sounds of drills.

Need help on your meditation journey? There's an app for that. *Calm, Headspace,* and *Insight Timer* are three of the most popular meditation apps. They provide a wide variety of guided meditations that teach you the history, process, and benefits of this practice. Give it a try - it's free!

The mental toll of the 40-hour (or 45-hour, 50-hour…) workweek should not be ignored. Small steps can help you reset your focus and approach your career with a clear mind. The sources of stress identified in this chapter can manifest into some serious physical and mental consequences. Physical and mental well-being are closely intertwined. Addressing one type of stress may alleviate stress in other areas. Stress lives in the body. By treating your body and mind right, you can take on the stress of any job, even dentistry.

Chapter 3:

Physical Toll of Practice

Take care of your body. It's the only place you have to live.
— **Eric Thomas**

Dentists are usually not surprised to hear that burnout is more prevalent among younger professionals. Pressure, high expectations, and chronic stress are mentally exhausting. I have barely even touched on the expectations that parents, friends, and partners may set years before dental school even begins. The national economy and society at large add their own pressure into the mix. But this generation is not the first to consider early retirement. Mental exhaustion isn't the only reason for early retirement, either. While some dentists are extending their careers to make ends meet, a large percentage of dentists are forced into early retirement due to physical exhaustion and even disability.

Forced early retirement has been present in the dental profession for decades. Studies trace this back to a handful of causes, including musculoskeletal disorders and cardiovascular disease. These disorders are often preventable. So why do some dentists still retire early?

Simply put, dentistry is a physically taxing profession. Dental school often glosses over practical education, like

71

ergonomics, that may help dentists adjust their posture and practice with physical health in mind. Perfect focus on surgery often takes priority to posture and physical safety. These physical demands fail to alleviate any of the mental stress associated with dentistry or related professions. If anything, they add to the stress. Stress prevents physical conditions from improving. Without proper education or awareness, professionals may create a cycle of discomfort and frustration.

In this chapter, we will look at the different ways in which the dental profession causes pain throughout the body. We will also dive deeper into the cycle of stress and discomfort, looking specifically at hypertension and a lack of sleep.

Don't stand all day at work? Not currently using a dental drill eight hours a day? You're not immune to physical pain at the office. You may still be at risk of back, neck, and shoulder problems. Long periods of sitting put you at a higher risk of stiff muscles and pain, regardless of where you're sitting. Increased screen time, both in and out of the workplace, also poses risks.

At the end of this chapter, I will provide a list of solutions and practices that can help you get back on your feet - without pain in the rest of your body. Do not let physical conditions put you on a path toward early retirement.

Time to Straighten Up

If you haven't noticed ads online for posture correctors, you will soon. Posture correctors, often in the form of back braces that fit under your clothes, are the hottest Amazon purchase for office workers. Do these products work as well as they claim? The research doesn't have a conclusive answer. In

2013, the National Institute of Health suggested that there is one obvious benefit of posture correctors: they make you aware of your posture. Simple self-awareness is proven to produce better posture and reduce the risk of developing musculoskeletal disorders.

Correcting your posture at work is often easier said than done. Dentists have to pay careful attention to their patients during exams or procedures. Sometimes our last priority can be maintaining good posture. Trying to sit up or stand up in a neutral position might become a distraction, or slow down surgery. Readjusting your focus every few seconds may cause mistakes. Plus, if no one is reminding you to straighten up, you're not going to make it a priority.

When I was a resident, I remember one of our attending faculty would attempt to "scare us straight". He would walk by anyone that was hunched over while in surgery and say, "This is where they're going to make the incision," while pointing to the spine. He was clearly indicating that we were on the trajectory towards back problems if we didn't "straighten up."

How Slouching Affects the Body

Slouching may feel "relaxed," but it puts a strain on very specific areas of the body. When the body slouches, the upper back, shoulders, and head reach forward. The head pulls the body farther forward, forcing the back to hold the body up. Normally, this is the job of the abdominal muscles. When slouched over, the abdominal muscles have no work to do, and they're being squished.

The spine takes on a lot of weight when the body is slouched over. Taking on this weight doesn't strengthen the back - it just puts it at risk of misalignment or strains. When you mess with the spinal cord, you mess with the entire central nervous system. Pain the shoulders, arms, and legs may trace back to misalignment or pinched nerves along the spine.

The spinal cord runs from the tailbone all the way up to the back of the head. Neck pain and back pain are closely related. Take a moment to feel how your body is positioned when you are hunched over your phone or twisting your back in a procedure. Your back may be misaligned, but the real problem lies in your neck. Serious strains in the neck are common not only in dentistry but also in other jobs that require proper posture.

Freezing your body in a slouched or twisted position puts pressure on nerves, vertebrae, and other areas of the body that quickly become fatigued. Repeating these twists and slouches, again and again, fatigues the body even faster. If posture is not corrected, real damage can be done.

Consequences of Slouching

Studies confirm how dangerous poor posture is for dentists and all professionals. Between 60-90% of dentists experience some form of musculoskeletal pain in their career, reporting higher rates of musculoskeletal disorders than medical professionals in other fields.

Disorders include, but are not limited to:

- Sprains and strains
- Pain in the back, neck, or shoulders
- Carpal tunnel syndrome
- Hernias and slipped discs

Experts at Brigham and Women's Hospital also warn professionals that poor posture can cause incontinence, heartburn, and constipation. It goes without saying that any of these conditions can make the workplace much more stressful.

Pain from slouching doesn't gradually become noticeable after decades in the field. In as little as three years, a majority of dentists report having some form of body pain. These disorders, if left untreated, can become severe. Up to 10% of people with musculoskeletal disorders become disabled. Remember, slouching and hunching over are preventable. These disorders are preventable.

Back pain and related musculoskeletal disorders force Americans to take over 264 million sick days per year. Treating larger conditions can take weeks or months. Correcting poor posture won't just make you look better at work - it will keep you able to practice for a longer period of time.

Unfortunately, poor posture is not the only threat to physical health in the world of dentistry.

I've Got to Hand It to You

When you picture a dentist performing a procedure, you might not see them twisting their spine or moving their entire body. Most of the body is frozen, with movement limited to the hands and wrists. Even the hands and wrists are barely moving as they focus on a small area of the mouth and make precise adjustments. These precise movements come with big consequences. Dentists face a high risk of hand and wrist injuries in addition to injuries around the spine and neck.

Wrist injuries? Hand injuries? Sure, dentists aren't engaged in sport, but they are moving their hands a lot. According to the

American Dental Association, any of the following movements or positions may aggravate or cause pain in the hands:

- Gripping tools tightly or statically for a long period

- Gripping tools with thin handles or vibrating pieces

- Repetitive motions

- Holding the wrist in a non-neutral position for a long period

Hand pain may originate, not just from how you're holding tools, but also from how intensely you are holding your tools.

ACTIVITY: Try this little exercise. Loosely grip the book or tablet you are holding. Now squeeze it as hard as you can! Harder! Squeeze!

There's a difference between those two grips, right? The pressure to perform well may cause you to grip your highspeed drill with more strength. A stronger grip exhausts the hands faster and puts you at a higher risk of strains and sprains. As you evaluate your posture throughout the day, evaluate the tension in your muscles and your grip on anything that you might be holding.

Eye Strain, You Strain

Hands are not the only body parts affected by the size of tools, teeth, and X-rays. Eye strain and trauma may also send a dentist into early retirement. Dentists have to see the smallest

76

details in order to perform procedures or spot a cavity. Sure, loupes help, but over time this near focus could cause a dentist's vision to weaken to the point where they can no longer practice safely. Not to mention, focusing on instruments and objects may also increase your risk of injury. Goggles and other eye protection can prevent irritants from entering the eye, but they can only do so much when you are squinting to pay attention to the tiny movements you are making with your hands.

Blood Pressure and High Stress

By now, we have established that the field of dentistry comes with a high amount of stress and anxiety. Stress does more than intensify the grip of your hands. Chronic stress can cause high blood pressure and more severe conditions. It affects the entire body.

Differentiating "chronic" stress from short-term stress is important when talking about the effects of pressures at work. In the short term, stress is tolerable. Humans have been experiencing stress since they first walked this earth. Predators, weather, and other stressors have always caused a reaction in the body. But the "predators" that we face now are much more prevalent than the predators in the past. Chronic stress, on the other hand, is harmful not only the cardiovascular but to other bodily systems, like muscular and nervous systems.

The Evolution of "Fight or Flight"

"Fight or flight" isn't just a phrase. It's a state of mind that even the earliest humans have faced. These humans weren't worried about student loans or what they heard on cable news. They were more worried about wild animals and warring tribes.

When early humans detected predators or other stressful situations, their brains put their bodies into action.

The "fight or flight" response prepared humans to either fight the stressor or run away to safety. Physiological responses involved in "fight or flight" include:

- Increased heart rate and contractility
- Constriction of the blood vessels
- Release of hormones, like adrenaline and norepinephrine

Our ability to fight or flee is elevated when our heart rate is elevated and certain hormones are released. "Fight or flight" was, and still can be a survival mechanism.

The "fight or flight" response to stress dies down when the source of stress is no longer present. Back in more primitive days, the body calmed down after humans escaped predators. Early humans then went back to their peaceful life of rest and digest. Nowadays, humans experience less leisure and more reasons to get stressed out. You know those moments when you are nervous about a meeting and your heart starts beating really fast? That's fight or flight. What about the stress of screwing up an extraction or root canal, which causes your palms to get sweaty? How about the stress of not having the experienced staff or assistants you need? Initiate fight or flight!

The occasional "fight or flight" response doesn't do too much damage to the body. But when you find yourself stressed out every day, the effects of this response linger. These effects include high blood pressure or hypertension.

Dangers of High Blood Pressure

Hypertension itself may not kill you instantly, but over time, it can damage arteries throughout the body. Again, the body is connected in ways that you might not expect.

High blood pressure is often the culprit behind the following conditions:

- Blocked arteries and heart attack
- Clogged arteries and strokes
- Heart failure
- Kidney failure
- Vision loss
- Narrowed arteries and pain throughout the body

High blood pressure seriously increases the risk of cardiovascular disease, the number one killer of dentists, Americans, and people around the world.

Eight out of ten cases of cardiovascular disease are preventable. Cardiovascular disease does not have to be the top killer of people in the world. It doesn't have to kill you, even if you are in a stressful job. Stress can take over your life and even take your life, but only if you let it. Healthy habits, including sleep and other forms of stress relief, can help to prevent the more dangerous effects of hypertension and a stressful job.

Trying to Sleep Can Be a Nightmare

All of these dangers can be stressful! Ironically for dentists, stress can cause people to have a dream that involves their teeth falling out. Some dentists can get so stressed that they don't even dream, or sleep, at all.

Stress and sleep are incompatible. Bodies do not go into "fight or flight or sleep" mode. If you are stressed about a patient, a treatment, or staff, you will have a harder time falling asleep. This cycle is dangerous for dentists *and* patients. Everyone needs a solid night of sleep to perform their best the next day. Without sleep, you are more likely to make mistakes - and put yourself at risk for serious health problems.

Why Is Sleep So Important, Anyway?

Sleep isn't just a cozy relief from work - it's an important way to reduce stress, recover from physical activity, and improve your overall well-being.

The body moves through different cycles of sleep at night. Each cycle has a checklist of tasks to help the body and mind process what happened earlier that day. These tasks include:

1. Reduction in blood pressure

2. Muscle and tissue repair

3. Release of human growth hormone

4. Appetite regulation

5. Memory storage

If you're stiff at the dental office all day, or you spent time at the gym, sleep is crucial for recovery and restoration. Lack of sleep can exaggerate the pain, strains, and misalignment caused by poor posture and repetitive motion at work.

You might know someone who brags about only getting two or four hours of sleep. Business leaders and celebrities sing the praises of people who spend more time in the office than in their bedroom. Don't let them fool you. You need sleep, and you need a full night's sleep to fully prepare for the next day.

Two, four, or six hours of sleep may not be enough to make a full recovery. Why? Sleep cycles move in a peculiar pattern. The body cycles in and out of light, deep, and REM sleep approximately every two hours. During this first cycle, the body enters REM sleep for one to five minutes at a time before moving onto other stages of sleep. As the body continues to rest, the time spent in deep or REM sleep lengthens. Four hours of sleep a night gives you significantly less time to regulate the body and prepare for a new day.

Sleep cycles include periods of light sleep or wakefulness. It's easier to transition out of sleep if you are in these stages than it is to wake up during REM sleep. If you wake up feeling refreshed after two or four hours of sleep, you might have just woken up while in these lighter stages. Aim for a full eight hours of sleep to get the REM sleep you need *and* wake up at the end of a sleep cycle. Apps like *Sleep Cycle* can help you achieve both of these goals.

Put the Phone Down

A full eight hours of sleep is crucial to getting a healthy amount of deep and REM sleep. Every minute tossing and turning holds you back from longer periods of rest and recovery. Like cardiovascular disease, a lot of tossing and turning is preventable. Insomnia and sleep problems aren't just the result of a stressful day. If you're saving your screen time for sundown, you could be putting yourself at risk for poor sleep.

It's tempting to look at your screen all day. Laptops allow us to chat with friends, watch Netflix, and pay bills from anywhere in the house. The whole world is in front of us, even if we're staring into a tiny screen. Late-night screen-time isn't just putting a strain on the eyes - it's keeping a lot of people up at night. Four in ten people admit to using their computer after 10 p.m. This habit can mess with your entire body.

A consistent workweek, like the 9-5, fits into the body's natural ability to stick to a routine. Bodies run on an internal, 24-hour clock. This clock, known as the circadian rhythm, influences our sleep-wake patterns. The release of hormones like melatonin, cortisol, and norepinephrine relies on this clock.

Like a traditional clock needs batteries, our internal clock needs cues from the environment to know what "time" it is. The biggest cue is light. Back in more primitive times, sunset would cue to the body to wind down. Melatonin would be released, and humans would ease into sleep. (Hormones do more than regulate our sleep-wake cycle. Norepinephrine, for instance, plays a role in regulating blood pressure. Lack of sleep and disrupted circadian rhythms increase the risk of hypertension and other cardiovascular conditions.)

Artificial lights like phones, computer screens, and eReaders disrupt our internal clocks. Bodies cannot tell the difference between light coming from the sun and light coming from an iPhone. Even if the room around you is dark, persistent exposure to the blue light from your phone may prevent you from going to sleep.

This creates an unfortunate cycle for anyone with a phone nearby. Before they go to bed, they check their phone. After an hour of tossing and turning, they might check their phone again, delaying sleep further. After another hour...you get the picture.

Recognizing this cycle, like recognizing poor posture, is the first step to correcting it. You do not have to live in cycles of stress, discomfort, and more stress. All it takes to break the cycle of insomnia and blue light exposure is to just get off your phone. Small adjustments can make a huge difference in your physical health and overall well-being. These adjustments could allow you to potentially practice in clinical dentistry longer and far better-off.

Let's Get Physical

Understanding the risks of musculoskeletal disorders, high blood pressure, and poor sleep can help you reduce yours. Consider any of the following solutions to improve posture, strength, and your overall physical health while navigating clinical dentistry:

√ Get adequate exercise throughout the day

√ Visit a chiropractor or masseuse

√ Learn more about ergonomics in the workplace

√ Change up your sleeping position

√ Prepare for sleep properly

√ Reconsider your workload

Adequate Exercise

As we adapt to poor posture, we lose strength in our back and other postural muscles. Our pectoral muscles lose flexibility, and our abdominal muscles weaken. Using good posture can help us regain this strength, but it can cause pain or fatigue in the office. Instead, prepare your body for good posture by exercising and stretching regularly. Build up your core and pectoral muscles. Strengthen your lower back and stabilize your pelvic muscles. It won't be so tiring to stand or sit up straight throughout the day if you commit to exercising.

Short, "micro workouts" can help you get your exercise in without spending an hour at the gym. Look up 10-minute HIIT (high intensity interval training) workouts or yoga flows that are designed to help your posture. Even a few one-minute planks throughout the day can build up strength in the muscles that need it. Working out can kill two birds with one stone by reducing symptoms of anxiety and depression. Counteract the mental and physical toll of your work with exercise! These "Micro workouts" can be a great way to burn some calories without breaking a sweat at work.

Don't Forget to Stretch!

You can even spend a few minutes each hour stretching. Stretching allows the muscles to build more strength and prevents stiffness from repetitive motions or standing still during surgery. If you are not stretching before and after a workout (or after a long procedure), consider adding a few to your routine.

You can find stretches for the back, neck, abdominals, and even the wrists and hands online. Stretch at the top of every hour or when you need a quick moment to relax and refocus. Who says dentists are stiff?

Health Insurance and Disability

Having proper health insurance or disability coverage provides protection from unsuspecting financial hardship due to a severe illness or injury and can provide you with peace of mind, knowing that you will still be able to support you and your family's current lifestyle. The ADA even offers plans that can pay benefits all the way to age 67. If you become completely disabled from being able to practice dentistry in a clinic setting, you'll get full benefits, even if you are able to work in another area of dental practice or choose to enter a new profession.

There are three factors insurance providers look at when deciding if you qualify for disability insurance:

1. **Health:** Do you have pre-existing conditions? Are you overweight? Do you smoke?

2. **Age:** The younger you are, the more likely you are to qualify due to less health issues you will typically have.

3. **Income:** The more money you make may give you the ability to purchase additional coverage.

Therefore, usually a good time to buy disability insurance is sooner rather than later. Be sure to find an insurance carrier that can determine what coverage is best for you and your family's future.

Get a Physical Therapist

If you have been injured in the past, you might be hesitant to go to the gym or start working out. That's okay! You can still get back into exercising with the help of a physical therapist. Physical therapists assess their patient's injuries, range of motion, and movement goals. (More PTs are providing telehealth services in light of COVID-19.) After an evaluation, therapists can provide exercises and workout routines customized to your needs, schedule, and workplace demands. They can also act as an "accountability buddy." You may be more likely to exercise if you have someone to answer to every month.

Visit a Chiropractor or Masseuse

Physical therapists are not the only people who can help dentists and professionals prevent physical injury. How does a monthly massage sound?

Massages do more than give you an excuse to go to the spa and treat yourself. A monthly massage can "undo" the stiff knots that are built up during long periods of standing during stationary or treatments. They loosen up muscles, increase flexibility, and enable you to recover faster. Studies from researcher and nurse, Christine Olney, show that massage therapy can also be an effective treatment for high blood pressure. Plus, who doesn't love an hour away from their phone, relaxing, and taking your mind off of work?

Spas aren't the only place where you can get a massage. If you have specific spinal issues, consider getting a chiropractic massage. Chiropractors often offer massage therapy that has a special focus on the spine and surrounding muscles. Similar to physical therapists, chiropractors can also help you recover from specific injuries. Look for chiropractors that specialize in back, neck, or even wrist pain. A single session can help you "reset" and send you back in the operatory with more mobility and less pain.

Understanding Ergonomics

Monthly visits to a professional are a great opportunity to get into the knots, nerves, and muscles that you can't reach yourself. Exercise can help you prepare for long hours of sitting or standing properly. But do you really know how to sit up correctly in your chair? Can you perform procedures without increasing your risk of back pain?

You spend more time at work than you do getting massages or working out at the gym. So, make sure you understand ergonomics and how to reduce the risk of pain at work.

Ergonomics is the study of increasing comfort and efficiency in the workplace. Proper posture and pain-free workdays allow employees to be more productive and saves companies millions of dollars in workers' compensation and paid medical leave. Straightening up at work is a win-win.

It's not enough to know that you *should* improve your posture. Ergonomics looks at how chairs and desks affect posture, and how to properly design an operatory for optimal efficiency. No, you don't have to redo your entire office to avoid back and neck pain. Proper lighting may be just as effective. The right magnifying tools, like loupes, can also help you clearly see your patient's mouth while keeping your neck in a neutral position. Seemingly small adjustments can provide serious pain relief.

If you are interested in applying the principles of ergonomics to your workplace, consider taking a course. Proper posture and ergonomic exercises can take up entire chapters, books, and anthologies. Courses are readily available on *YouTube*, OSHA's website, or through top-level universities. You do not have to get a certification to learn how to improve your posture and enhance your workspace. Even the basics can make a big difference.

ACTIVITY. Try to follow these ergonomic rules next time you're in the operatory.

- √ Use magnification and illumination
- √ Correct working length from eye to patient
- √ Neck flexion no more than 20°
- √ Upper body leaning forward less than 20°
- √ Shoulders relaxed
- √ Upper arms rotated forward 10° - 20°
- √ Elbows tucked in at sides
- √ Forearms inclined upwards 0° - 25°
- √ Back support at upper pelvis
- √ Back straight
- √ Hips higher than knees
- √ Chair raised to create ~ 110° angle behind knee
- √ Legs spread slightly apart at no more than 45°
- √ Lower legs perpendicular to the floor
- √ Both feet flat on the floor

Sleeping Positions

Poor posture isn't limited to the dental office. The way that you sit at home, and the way that you sleep at night, could exaggerate problems with posture or back pain. Changing the way you sleep may be uncomfortable at first, but will benefit your posture and overall pain levels in the long run.

The healthiest sleep position for your posture is one of the least popular: sleeping on your back. Sleeping on your back (with a supportive pillow) allows your head, neck, and spine to rest in a neutral position throughout the night. This is almost impossible when you sleep on your stomach.

While sleeping on your back may be ideal for most, it is unhealthy for others. If you snore, you'll snore louder while sleeping on your back. In this case, it might be best to sleep on your side. Side sleepers may be able to rest in a neutral position if they use pillows correctly. (A supportive pillow and a pillow between the knees can prop up the head and neck while taking the curve out of the spine.)

Preparing for Sleep

If your mind is racing before bed, you're going to have trouble staying in healthy sleeping positions. Stop tossing and turning for hours before you get to sleep. Simple tips like these can help you get to sleep faster and get the most out of your time in bed.

√ **Reduce blue light.** Put your phones in a separate room or on the "Do Not Disturb" mode. Swap out tablets for books. Once you have separated yourself from blue light for an hour, your body will start to produce melatonin and ease into sleep naturally.

89

√ **Reserve your bed for sleeping.** If you do find yourself tossing and turning, head into another room. Your bed should not be a place for worrying or overthinking. Dim the lights, read a book, and only go back to your room when you're ready to sleep.

√ **Take a hot (or cold) shower before bed.** The choice is yours. A hot shower or bath can help loosen up the muscles and calm the mind. But there are advantages in a cold shower, too. When the body begins to transition into sleep, its core temperature drops. Cold showers aid in that transition. Plus, any worries that you have before bed will immediately go away when you enter a cold shower.

Reconsider Your Workload

A warm bubble bath and two hours without blue light may not have an impact if your mind is constantly going back to your treatments, caseload, and frustrating patients. If you are having trouble sleeping, keep track of how often work leaves you tossing and turning. Do you want to let your workload put you at risk of hypertension and sleep deprivation?

Do not forget about sleep when you are weighing your career options. A high salary may not make up for nights tossing and turning. Lack of sleep comes with a cost.

■■

If you are stressed out by your job, it might be time to reconsider your position and the workload that you take on each day.

■■

90

You have a lot of opportunities to make your day at work easier to manage and more comfortable. Mental and physical obstacles will always be in your way as you work. Sitting, standing, dealing with management, and handling finances will always be part of the job. But small solutions, like the ones described in this chapter and previous chapters, can alleviate the stress and pressure working long hours in the operatory.

In the following chapters, we will begin to look at the changes that have shaped the workweek in the past, present, and post-COVID world. The 9-5 doesn't look the same as it did in 2000, 1990, or 1880. As our world evolves, more opportunities become available to professionals in every field. These opportunities could be the solution to finding a career away from clinical dentistry that you enjoy, developing a schedule that fits your lifestyle, and discovering a life that allows you to live out your passions.

Part II

How We Got Here

Chapter 4:

The Overtime Dentist

No one on his deathbed ever said, 'I wish I had spent more time at the office.'.

— Paul Tsongas

When I first began shadowing other dentists, I was drawn to the "perks" of being able to create my own schedule. Dentists could stay in business and enjoy a decent salary without working five days a week. Marketing costs were close to zero - there was little competition in the dental field and everyone needed a dentist. Office rent was cheap, too. The dentists I shadowed had little to no student loan debt, so their salary only needed to cover the basic costs of living.

A dentist could work four days a week without many complaints. Dentists who didn't need a hefty salary could get away with working three full days and a few extra hours here and there. This flexibility appealed to a lot of my colleagues. I mean, who *doesn't* want to avoid the old "9 to 5?"

Through a recent global pandemic and advances in computer technology have given many professionals the "freedom" to avoid the traditional workweek. In the next chapter, I will address the attitudes and opportunities that are allowing more people to have flexible schedules. But before I talk about leaving the 9 to 5 of dentistry, I want to discuss how these two hours became the expectations for your day, week, and life.

"Workin' 9 to 5"

The average workday starts at 9 a.m., ends at 5 p.m., and lasts Monday through Friday. You get weekends off, and most holidays if you're lucky. It's so ingrained in our culture, there are even hit songs and movies simply called "9 to 5."

9 to 5 is commonplace, but not something that most people appreciate or dream about. Just take a look at some of the lyrics to Dolly Parton's "9 to 5:"

"Workin' 9 to 5, what a way to make a livin'
Barely gettin' by, it's all takin' and no givin'
They just use your mind and they never give you credit
It's enough to drive you crazy if you let it
9 to 5, for service and devotion
You would think that I would deserve a fat promotion
Want to move ahead but the boss won't seem to let me
I swear sometimes that man is out to get me!"

Dolly Parton isn't talking about dentists when she performs this song, although the lyrics are certainly relatable. One could argue that "9 to 5" could apply to everyone in the dentist's office, from the receptionists to the owner of the practice to the patients who are taking the afternoon off to make their appointment.

NPR called this song a "workers' anthem across decades," despite (and because of) the dissatisfaction expressed by Parton. "9 to 5" encapsulates many of the issues that workers across the country feel, despite being in different industries: rising cost of living, pressure from upper management, lack of

95

recognition, and devoting yourself to a career that leaves you unfulfilled.

It's no surprise that many Americans find themselves devoting more hours a week to work. We feel as though staying late, arriving early, and producing more will result in the recognition and fulfillment Parton longs for in her song. Of course, when every other employee is *also* staying late and working early, we don't get that recognition and fulfillment. Why should anyone be considered special when everyone else is clocking in for 45 or 50 hours a week? When a 40-hour (minimum) workweek is all that millennials, Gen X'ers, and Baby Boomers have ever known, how can you be expected to *leave* it for something shorter?

The answer may lie in the history of the 9-5, and how it affects the way that everyone attempts to plan out their week of work, recreation, and rest. You might be surprised to learn that a 9-5 workday was once considered "revolutionary" in American history. People fought, sometimes losing their lives, for the right to only work 40 hours a week.

■■■

As dentists we find ourselves working more than 40 hours most weeks when you total everything up.

■■■

Working overtime is not an act intended to counter what was once revolutionary. Instead, we are putting in over 40 hours a week *just* to see and treat patients, satisfy upper management, or pay bills and debts.

In this chapter, I will go over the past, present, and future of working 9-5, both in the United States and around the world. When you look at the data, you might be surprised to learn that Americans put in more hours than most developed nations, often *at the expense* of productivity. This data urges Americans in all professions to fight for a change, both at a national level and within their own industries. These changes are starting to take place. By using the tips provided at the end of this chapter, you can begin to make a change for yourself, your colleagues, and anyone feeling the dissatisfaction of a *9 to 5.*

How Did We Get Here?

Forty hours may be an overwhelming schedule for many, but it would have been considered a relief from the weekly schedule for laborers in the early days of America. In the early 1800s, laborers were expected to work close to 16 hours a day. Some even clocked in a whopping 100 hours each week. (Talk about no work-life balance.) Welsh labor rights activist Robert Owen is credited for spearheading the 8-hour workweek we know today. He called for "Eight hours work, eight hours recreation, eight hours rest."

Inspired by the labor movement happening across the pond, American workers began calling for a ten-, and later eight-hour workday. Protests calling for an eight-hour workday erupted around the country. In 1886, protesters gathered at Haymarket Square in Chicago to support workers who were striking for an eight-hour work week. The protest, now known as the Haymarket Square Riot, ended in gunfire. At least eight people died while fighting for a 40-hour workweek.

The private sector finally listened and started to enact forty-hour work weeks, following the lead of Henry Ford. Ford was one of the first business owners to encourage a five-day workweek for his employees. He said,

"Just as the eight-hour day opened our way to prosperity in America, so the five-day workweek will open our way to still greater prosperity. It is high time to rid ourselves of the notion that leisure for workmen is either lost time or a class privilege."

Twenty years after Ford made the five-day workweek popular, Congress put it into law. The Fair Labor Standards Act stated that any time over 40 hours a week was "overtime." As a result of this law, 700,000 Americans saw an increase in pay and a reduction in hours. The Fair Labor Standards Act has been amended many times since it was passed in the 1930s and is still the law that oversees minimum wage and overtime pay today. Although small changes have been made to minimum wage, a strict 40-hour workweek remains as the standard throughout the country.

Of course, the rules of overtime pay set by the Fair Standards Labor Act don't apply to everyone, including most dentists. Executive, administrative, and professional employees who earn a yearly salary or commission/production-based pay are not covered by the FLSA. Independent contractors are not covered. If you make your own hours, you are not covered. The failure to protect these workers leaves many Americans vulnerable to the pressures of the market, company culture, and general anxiety around productivity. Despite the "standard" work week set at 40 hours, many dentists find themselves working overtime *without* overtime pay.

How Dentists Started Working the 9-5

The Fair Labor Standards Act does not apply to dentists who want to open up their own practice and make their own schedule. (Dentists who are business owners *should* consider fair labor practices when determining the schedules and pay of their receptionists, hygienists, etc., but for now, let's talk about dentists themselves.)

This exclusion has never mattered much to dentists. Dentists in the "Golden Age of Dentistry" probably considered the traditional 40 hours-a-week schedule to be working *overtime*. No one opened up their own practice with the intention of working 9 to 5. They wanted to avoid the tediousness of clocking in and clocking out like everyone else. Three or four days with a shortened schedule was the "standard" for dentists in recent decades.

Dentists set these standards because they *could*. All an individual practice needed to do was cover rent, operating costs, and drum up a satisfactory salary for the owner. And when you think about the costs of dental procedures, covering every expense could be done by seeing only a few patients a week. Keeping up with the costs of operating was "easy" for dentists 10, 20, or 30 years ago. Now, some dentists are seriously struggling. Rent prices have gone up dramatically. With more dentists in the area, many have to spend money on marketing or increase operating costs to stand out. Many providers will buy the latest technology in order to compete with the fancy dental office down the street. For many new practice owners, a decision is made whether to pay yourself more or put it back in the dental practice.

Yet, dentists need to make a higher salary than ever before. The costs of dental school add a significant amount of money to a dentist's monthly expenses. If you've racked up $500,000 in student loans, you're going to need to pay a minimum of $2,000 or $3,000 just to pay them off in *30 years*.

This adds significant pressure to dentists to stay open and accept more patients. It's not sustainable to go to dental school, take on the costs of running your own practice, and work three or four days a week.

In recent years, dentists have had to abandon the idea that working 9-5 was overtime. An increasing number of dentists are working five, six, or seven days a week. These hours may include nights and weekends, just to become more accessible to patients. (Part 2 of this book goes into more detail about the investments that dentists must make in order to maintain a private practice or simply practice as a dentist.)

Dentists aren't just working more than 4 days a week in 2020 - they're starting to work *true* overtime hours. These extra hours may bring in more cash, but they're not growing private practices or DSOs at any significant higher rate. A rise in self-made dental practice consultants has risen over the years, all claiming they have the answer to this large problem in dentistry. They all offer you their "secret" to getting more patients and making more money while working less. However, as I've mentioned before, these "secrets" can come at a high price.

Where Do We Stand in the World?

It's not just dentists who find themselves working longer hours. In 2018, the Organization for Economic Cooperation and Development collected data from developed and developing nations around the world to assess the "average" workweek. While Americans certainly don't work as many hours as countries like Mexico or Korea, we still work more hours on average than most of the developing world.

The average employee in the countries surveyed works 1,760 hours each year. That comes down to 33.8 hours per week, including the weeks that employees spend on vacation or celebrating holidays. Americans work an average of 1,780 hours each year. Compare this number to countries like Germany, who work an average of 1,360 hours each year. At the end of 2017, the average employee in the United Kingdom worked 1,680 hours each year, or 32.3 hours per week.

No Such Thing as Paid Time Off

Like most dentists, there's no such thing as having any paid time off (PTO). All vacations or time away from the clinic is time that you do not receive any compensation. When a dental provider wants to take time off not only does he or she have to dig in his savings to afford to take time off, he or she also has to prepare for the lack of production as a result of their trip. This is if your company or private practice even lets you have the wanted time away. Some DSOs will limit the number of days you request away from the office, for fear of not making budget and production goals. Not only do issues occur over vacations or holidays but also sick days and maternity/paternity leaves.

■■■

The last thing you want to think when your child is born is 'when should I return to work?

■■■

Meanwhile, many current careers, especially in the tech industry, are offering complete paid time off with the possibility of working from home or any destination of your choosing.

When we compare the United States and the United Kingdom, it is also important to note that *other* federal policies impact when employees in each respective country are working. Sure, many Americans who are paid hourly can get "time and a

101

half" for working over 40 hours a week. But we pale in comparison when it comes to paid holidays, sick days, and other types of leave. Paid holidays and maternity leave are a right, not a privilege, in the United Kingdom and most developed nations. The United States is the only developed country without a federal law mandating paid vacation or maternity leave. The United Kingdom offers 28 days of paid vacation for every employee each year. France offers 30 *and* one paid holiday. Over a dozen other countries offer 20 days of paid vacation.

The average worker took 17 days of vacation, which is still less than what other developed countries *require* workers to take each year. After spending years in school to become a dentist, while some of your non-dental friends and family were able to travel and take plenty of vacations, you deserve to take whatever time you need in order to be a content and productive human being.

No Vacation = No Work-Life Balance

Vacation is more than just a chance to be "lazy" or "do nothing." Having a career where you are still able to take vacation days while being compensated, provide people the opportunity to travel, explore hobbies, and spend time with their family. Robbing yourself (or your family) of that time only tips the scales of an already unhealthy work-life balance. Despite dentists *wanting* a work-life balance, the pressure to work long and hard pervades into every industry and job position in the country. If your friends, associates, or colleagues are not taking vacation time, you might ask yourself, why should you?

ACTIVITY: How does your work-life balance stack up? Answer TRUE or FALSE to assess how clinical dentistry is affecting your work-life balance.

— I am practicing dentistry and/or thinking about dentistry more than 40 hours a week.

— I usually see patients and skip a lunch break.

— I always research dental topics outside of business hours.

— I feel like I have no control over ability to give high-quality care to patients.

— I frequently feel frustrated or anxious due to staff, equipment, patients, or scheduling.

— I often feel guilty because I can't make time for everything I want to do.

— My family often complains about how stressed I am due to practicing dentistry.

— Sometimes I feel as though I've lost sight of who I am and why I chose dentistry.

— I've lost control of my temper while at work on multiple occasions.

— I can't remember the last time I took an extended vacation.

— I've missed important family events because of I wanted to provide access to care for patients.

— Dentistry leaves me feeling physically and emotionally exhausted.

Are you finding that you are answering more TRUE than FALSE? If so, it's time to take some control back in how you practice and life your life.

Productivity Determines Schedule Changes

Even as dentists, we are pressured to see more patients and increase the number of treatments to make up for the time off we want to take. Why do we feel pressured to stay at work longer in the first place? It's the same reason why Henry Ford initially reduced the workweek at Ford Motor Company to 40 hours: productivity. We want to get more work done each day so that we can make more money each day. We want our businesses to grow. Dentists want their practices to take on more patients, to charge those patients higher prices, and to turn a higher profit that will later go back into opening a larger space or more offices. Corporations that own dental practices are even *more* driven to grow the practices that they own. If they can maximize productivity *without* increasing costs, they find themselves in a pretty good place.

In order to increase productivity, Henry Ford didn't just *decrease* the workweek to 40 hours. He also *doubled* the pay of his employees. Before 1914, employees at Ford Motor Company were working nine hours a day for $2.34 an hour. (This was standard across the industry.) After Ford's changes, workers made $5 an hour, working eight hours a day. This boosted productivity throughout Ford Motor Company.

Ford also believed that reducing the workweek from six days to five days would increase productivity. When the changes were made, Henry Ford's son told the New York Times:

"Every man needs more than one day a week for rest and recreation... The Ford Company always has sought to promote [an] ideal home life for its employees. We believe that in order to live properly every man should have more time to spend with his family."

The extra money earned by employees was also encouraged to go out into the market, boosting the economy as well as productivity.

Very rarely do we see CEOs or private practice owners reducing hours *and* giving out 100% raises to increase growth and productivity. Nowadays, employers sing a different tune. We glorify business leaders who put in over 40 hours of work a week. We equate longer hours, more patients, busier schedules with more stamina, determination, and grit. If we want to prove to an employer that we are dedicated, we have to work until late in the night.

■■

Don't get me wrong, working hard in itself is not a bad thing.

■■

Putting in long hours for something you are passionate about and enjoy doing (while being able to give attention to other aspects of your life) is great. It's when we are working hard for someone else's goal or for reasons that don't give us purpose and joy – that is when it becomes problematic. Working long hours on personal goals when done appropriately increases your chance of success in the thing you want to be successful at. If being in the dental office 5-6 days a week from sun up to sundown gives you pleasure, then by all means toss this book in the trash.

Elon Musk tweeted that it takes 80-100 hours of work each week to "change the world," bragging to reporters that he logged up to 120 hours a week during the production of the Tesla Model 3. When Bill Gates reflects on his early years at Microsoft, he says, "I didn't believe in weekends; I didn't believe in vacations." Gates is rumored to also log up to 120 hours of work each week. Colleagues say that Gates also "drove others as hard as he drove himself." Gates and Musk are not anomalies, but they are role models for other leaders. Tesla and Microsoft are far from the only companies that pressure employees to work longer hours. Harvard Business Review followed 27 CEOs, who worked an average of 9.7 hours each day. When employers see their CEOs staying late, they are often pressured to do the same.

The USA's "Special Century"

The "special century" is a term in Robert J. Gordon's *The Rise and Fall of American Growth* used to describe the century following the Civil War. This 100-year period is so special because it shows a tremendous amount of growth - one that arguably put our country in the position that led many Americans to boast that "we're number one." As you'll remember from the beginning of this chapter, the "special century" begins just as Americans were beginning to fight for a 40-hour workweek.

Growth and productivity were not cut short due to fewer working hours. In fact, the contrary occurred. Gordon said that between 1870 and 1970, a "singular interval of rapid growth that will not be repeated." This growth can be partially credited to modern innovations, ranging from the Mason Jar to the electric freezer, yet these products were invented, sold, and distributed throughout the country as the modern workweek decreased in hours. Not only did this "special century" decrease the amount of hours worked per week, *but* it also decreased the amount of hours worked in a lifetime.

The first use of the term "weekend" did not appear until 1879. Retirement was not possible for many Americans until the Social Security Act was passed in 1935. Even then, retirement began at age 65, and the life expectancy for men and women was 58 and 62, respectively. Spending your golden years golfing is a concept that is fresher than that of the 40-hour workweek.

Not So Special Anymore

The "special century" ended 50 years ago and a lot has changed. We have the Internet, smartphones, self-driving cars, and other modern conveniences that make it easy to communicate, connect, and complete everyday tasks. According to Gordon, this hasn't allowed us to push forward any faster than in the early 1900s. Productivity has increased, but not significantly.

"[Total Factor Productivity] grew after 1970 at barely a third the rate achieved between 1920 and 1970."

Increased hours at work have not helped us, either.

The 1970s also marked a shift in how employers view the 40-hour workweek. In the late 1970s, Americans were working the same amount of hours as most Europeans. This has since changed. The American workweek began to slowly increase after 1979. Now, we clock in over 100 more hours each year, without much growth to show for it. Gordon says "western Europe and Japan largely caught up to the United States in the second half of the twentieth century." Are longer hours really the answer to growth and productivity? Gordon, along with many experts, would argue that it's not. I have had several colleagues, including myself, proclaim that they have increased their income since cutting back days. It's time to consider if you are more productive the more days you work or if it's time to make an adjustment.

Remember to assess your situation and note that the grass may not be greener leaving dentistry either. Many careers can be subjected to long hours. The important thing is that you feel fulfilled and supported in the thing you are doing.

Longer Hours Leads to a Loss in Productivity

It's easy to get lost in the large scale of centuries and nations. Let's zoom in to the individual, who rarely becomes more productive once they have logged in 40 hours each week.

Dentists need to pay serious attention to their patients while they are working. You don't want to miss a diagnosis or lose focus during a cavity preparation. A simple mistake can result in a bad review, lawsuits, or further damage to patients in the long run. Teeth are nothing to mess around with. Does it make sense, then, to work until you collapse? No. Working until exhaustion doesn't make sense for *anyone*.

Experts recommend that adults get eight hours of sleep a night. This number is not just pulled from Robert Owen's idea of "eight hours work, eight hours recreation, eight hours rest." Eight hours of sleep allows the body to move through light, deep, and REM sleep stages multiple times. These different stages of sleep allow the body and mind to reset. Critical hormones, like the human growth hormone and cortisol, are released during sleep. Without a good night's sleep, you increase your risk of feeling groggy and foggy during the day. No one wants a dentist who is consistently "groggy and foggy."

108

Sleep deprivation has a *serious* impact on productivity, and increased hours at work are costing American businesses a lot of money. How much? Researchers at Harvard University predict that insomnia costs the average American worker 11.3 days' worth of productivity each year. Converted to dollars, that's a whopping $63.2 billion. That money would forgive a lot of dentists facing six figures in student loan debt. Sleep is more valuable than you might think.

Despite pressure from management, the practice owner, or the larger American culture, working more than 4 days a week as a dentist does not make someone more productive or "worthy" as a provider. The dentists that know this have begun to make a change in their lives and their practice. There are plenty of providers who make the same (if not more) since working less days rather than more.

Mindtools.com states that productivity is typically comprised of five different elements organization, attitude, delegation, information integration, and effective use of systems.

ACTIVITY: In determining how productive you are, check off the below statements that applies to you.

— I delegate appropriate tasks to others to work more efficiently.

— I organize my day to take advantage of natural highs and lows in my energy and motivation.

— I actively look for ways to improve the flow of my work, and the way that I approach tasks.

— I can maintain focus on one task for a significant period of time.

— I spend lots of time looking for information or documents, or locating missing items.

— I actively look for ways to avoid wasting time and effort - both for myself and for my team.

— I multitask.

— I use the talents, time, and expertise of other people on my team to help get the work done.

— I use techniques like skimming and note taking to identify the key points from the documents that I receive.

— I use a formal tracking system to understand how I spend my time.

— I have a clear plan for dealing with disruptions and interruptions.

— The volume of correspondence and documentation that I receive on a daily basis overwhelms me.

— I delay difficult or unpleasant tasks until the last minute - or until the issue disappears on its own.

— To ensure that things are done right, I keep close track of the activities and decisions of others on my team.

— I find that my mind wanders, and it's hard to concentrate for long.

— I do all of the tasks that are assigned to me, and hope that I can keep up with the volume of work.

Are there areas in dentistry or life that you could be more productive? You might find that by changing your actions and mindset, you can avoid spending more time at the dental office and be just as productive (if not more)!

The Future of the 9-5

Americans in the 1800s fought for a 40-hour workweek. Some even lost their lives. But the cries for revolution during this time have since been drowned out by the pressure to be more productive and dedicate more time to work. In recent decades, many Americans have lost sight of how important it is to get "eight hours work, eight hours recreation, eight hours rest." Others simply cannot afford to clock out at 5 p.m. Student loans do not stop racking up interest when you go home at night.

Fortunately, dentists are starting to see how a longer workweek can cause physical, mental, and emotional damage. The data I have presented in this chapter is just a fraction of what dental providers are starting to see and use as leverage to negotiate terms and change industry culture. Although change may not happen in your office, it is happening. The future of 9-5 may not be one where everyone is "barely gettin' by."

Globalization, technology, and even the recent COVID-19 pandemic are providing more opportunities for employers to negotiate terms and create a healthier work-life balance. "Digital nomads" are taking their remote jobs to the farthest corners of the Earth to reduce the cost of living and enjoy a more relaxed lifestyle. Disciples of Tim Ferris' *The Four-Hour Workweek* are starting businesses to fund their lifestyles through a passive income. The opportunities are endless, even if you have a degree in a specific field. It *is* possible to enjoy a healthy work-life balance. It *is* possible to keep your job and still enjoy up to a month of vacation each year. The digital nomad lifestyle or a flexible schedule is not just accessible to a handful of tech superstars.

As you are probably well aware, you are in a field that is unable to break away from being at the office.

■■■

As new industries expand and utilize technology, you
might start to contemplate switching careers to obtain
the work-life balance you desire and deserve.

■■■

However, if the solution is to just leave dentistry part-
time, then active steps will need to be taken still.

What Can You Do?

Change starts with the individual. By recognizing the
risks of overworking yourself, you can reprioritize your schedule
and reassess your expectations. A healthy work-life balance is
possible in every industry, including dentistry. You won't
achieve it until you take action.

Understand Your "Why."

Action may begin with assessing your current position.
How many hours are you really working each week? How many
of those hours are considered productive? If you find yourself
spending more than 40 hours at the dental office, ask yourself
why.

We have gone over a few of the reasons why dentists stay at their jobs over time:

- Pressure from upper management

- A practice that equates longer hours or more days with more production

- Wanting a practice partnership, raise, or extra benefits

- Rising cost of living and/or high debt

Many dentists use these reasons as excuses to stay at work for 5, 6, or even 7 days a week. Yet, an unhealthy work-life balance and pressure to stay in the office accounts for two of the reasons why many dentists are dissatisfied with their careers.

Once you figure out why you are staying at the office longer, you need to take action to address those issues and begin to scale back to a "normal" 40-hour workweek (or something shorter!)

Negotiate Your Terms

Renegotiating your terms may be all it takes to achieve satisfaction. I will provide more detailed guidance on reassessment and renegotiation tactics in Chapter 9 of this book. Although it feels uncomfortable to ask for more money, it is less uncomfortable than staying stagnant for one, two, or ten more years.

The knowledge throughout this book, including the history outlined in this chapter, can help you as you renegotiate. If you perform better *after* your vacation, rather than before, be

113

sure to share this with your employer. An increase in pay is likely to lead to a reduction in stress and a boost in productivity. If this is all you need, ask for it.

Talk to Your Coworkers

Of course, renegotiating your terms is usually easier said than done. Insecurities may get in the way of confronting your boss and asking for a raise. Another roadblock may be a lack of knowledge. If you do not know how much your colleagues are getting paid, you may not know whether your requests are "unreasonable" or whether they will bring you up to speed with everyone around you.

Discussions about salary have long been considered "taboo." No one is expected to share how much money they make, especially with colleagues who work for the same company. It feels scandalous to even think about asking another dentist how much they make or what percentage of production/collections they receive. If you work with other associate dentists then this could be a great opportunity to gather information about pay in your office. Although it may be considered distasteful, discussing your salary is protected by federal law. The National Labor Relations Act of 1935 protects employees who want to discuss salary. (Specifically, the law protects any "concerted activities for the purpose of collective bargaining or other mutual aid or protection.") Pay secrecy policies are not only discouraged, they are often illegal. This does not cover independent contractors, but still covers more workers than the policies enacted in the Fair Standards Labor Act.

Do not be afraid to talk to dentists in your office or old classmates about what percentage of collections they are receiving. Knowledge is power. Be transparent with your dissatisfaction, even if you are embarrassed. Embarrassment may be a sign that you need to ask for more money.

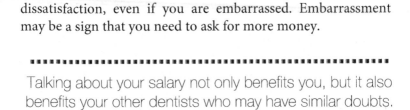

Talking about your salary not only benefits you, but it also benefits your other dentists who may have similar doubts.

If these discussions result in higher wages and increased productivity, one could argue that "everyone wins."

Lower Your Expectations for Immediate Change

These steps to renegotiate your situation may benefit you personally but are unlikely to promote rapid change throughout the field of dentistry. The culture surrounding modern-day dentists holds a tight grip on the minds of employers, providers, and leaders throughout the country. Although reading this book may allow you to reassess your priorities and fight for a shorter workweek, you are likely to meet opposition along the way.

Do not expect every colleague or employer to feel the same way that you feel. It took Bill Gates decades (and plenty of success) for him to walk back his original feelings about an 80- to 120-hour workweek. When leaders like Elon Musk are still praising a 100-hour work week, it feels hard to argue that scaling back is truly the solution. This misalignment is not a sign that you are unmotivated, lazy, or not dedicated enough to your work. You might just be working for the wrong employer, in the wrong position, or the wrong industry.

Chapter 5:

Where Do We Go from Here?

Work is a rubber ball. If you drop it, it will bounce back. The other four balls – family, health, friends, integrity – are made of glass. If you drop one of these, it will be irrevocably scuffed, nicked, perhaps even shattered.

– Gary Keller

The 9-5 has been a staple of American culture for decades, but fortunately, its foundations are crumbling. Technology, economics, and a global pandemic have forced business leaders to rethink where and when their employees work. The future of the "9-5" might not be bound to any time or location at all!

COVID-19 plays a big role in the future of the 9-5, especially in the world of dentistry. The global pandemic required dental offices to shut down for a period, but office rent was still due at the end of every month. Bills began to pile up, and the staff that *did* get paid were considered lucky. Patients were not quick to come back to the dentist, for fear of infection or *they* had less income to spare on treatments. After a few months, private practices contemplated selling their practices at a discount or to interested DSOs.

The inevitable shift toward corporate dentistry has been the push for *many* dentists to reconsider their career in the first place. If you are stepping away from the world of clinical dentistry, the "new normal" has many options for you to work not only in a new field but from anywhere in the world. If you have ever considered remote work or location independence, now is the time to start exploring your options.

Planning to stay in your current position? Dentists, surgeons, and other health professionals may shrug off the remote work revolution, claiming that the nature of their job makes it "impossible" to work remotely. But health professionals will not be left unaffected by the disruptions and innovations happening today. Now is the time to observe what is happening to the average worker, adapt, and see where *your* future fits into the future of the working world.

Whether you plan to stay in the dental industry, or plan to make a pivot in the next few years, understand the benefits and possibilities that come with remote work. Remote work is more accessible than ever before - and not for the reasons you might think.

COVID-19 Has Shown More Employers That Remote Work Is Possible

The COVID-19 pandemic flipped employment in America on its head. Tens of millions of people lost their jobs within a few weeks. Americans who were able to keep their jobs fell into one of two groups. One group was considered "essential workers," and stayed in the hospitals, grocery stores, and pharmacies where they had worked previously. The other group was sent home.

Before the Coronavirus pandemic, only a sliver of the population worked from home. Remote work seemed like a luxury, given to programmers in the tech world or employees with "open-minded" bosses. COVID-19 changed everything. Surveys say that between ⅓ and ⅔ of employed Americans are working from home.

Tech giants led the way in the remote work revolution. Amazon, Apple, and Twitter were some of the first companies to send their employees home in the wake of the pandemic. Facebook even sent remote employees $1,000 to help with expenses related to working from home. As the months crept on, companies like Facebook and Twitter *also* led the way in telling employees that they could continue working from home - forever. A career alternative that offers remote work is certainly appealing to dentists worried about the future COVID-19 infections.

Why Are Employers Offering Remote Work Now?

Social media platforms aren't the only companies that have embraced the idea of working from home indefinitely. Insurance companies, banks, and other businesses have decided to extend their work-from-home orders.

Part of these extended orders could be credited to the uncertainty surrounding the COVID and the development of a vaccine. On the other hand, employers were forced to let their employees work from home - and found that things were actually okay.

When Satya Nadella was asked about COVID-19's impact on the working world, the Microsoft CEO said "We have seen two years' worth of digital transformation in two months. From remote teamwork and learning to sales and customer service, to critical cloud infrastructure and security, we are working alongside customers every day to help them stay open for business in a world of remote everything. There is both immediate surge demand and systemic, structural changes across all of our solution areas that will define the way we live and work going forward."

Before COVID-19, employers refused to entertain the idea of working from home. Their reasons varied but could be traced back to a bit of stubbornness and contentment with current practices.

Here are some of the top reasons why managers, employers, and leaders refused to offer remote work:

1. Teams would be unmanageable without face-to-face interaction

2. No one would be able to see who is "on the clock," staying late, or arriving early

3. Switching to remote work would increase expenses

4. One employee switching to remote work would employ a domino effect, and soon everyone would demand remote work

5. Employees traditionally work in the office

6. Horror stories from select companies "prove" that remote work doesn't work

These horror stories often come from companies who tried to let employees work remotely *before* the technology was available to help them. Productivity and collaboration apps like *Slack* and *Zoom* weren't so popular before COVID-19. Now, every employee and their colleague use both platforms regularly.

119

Communication technology and other strategies have also helped employers manage their teams without physically being together. Strategies on management are easier to find now that more companies need help navigating the world of working remotely. Remote work was always possible. The COVID-19 just forced many companies to try it out. Now that they've taken the plunge, business leaders are starting to see that the water's fine.

Employees Are Happy to Work from Home

The truth is, while COVID-19 merely sped up the process of the remote work revolution. *FlexJobs* states that remote work grew 159% between 2005 and 2017. The majority of business leaders, however, were still not ready to embrace the future of working from home.

Experts believe that COVID-19 was the shake that some companies needed to let go of their stubborn views on remote work. Sure, there are drawbacks to working from home. Later in this chapter, I will touch on some of these drawbacks and how they might factor into decisions about working from home. But the data surrounding remote work suggests that it's not only cost-effective for employers - it's also more fulfilling for employees.

Take the company *Buffer*, for instance. *Buffer* offers social media management tools which service over 70,000 customers - with just 85 employees. *Buffer* is a pioneer in offering remote work and flexible schedules to their employees.

In 2020, they sent out a State of Remote Work Survey to over 3,500 employees who are working from home. They found that 98% of the remote workers who answered the survey would like to continue working remotely. 97% would recommend it to others.

Some of the advantages of working from home include:

- Ability to have a flexible schedule
- Flexibility to work from anywhere
- Not having to commute
- Ability to spend time with family

These advantages truly perk up the ears of college graduates and employees around the world. The ability to have a flexible schedule, for example, drew many of my colleagues into the world of dentistry. A flexible schedule usually gives you more time to spend with your family. If you time your hours right, you don't have to commute very far to your practice.

Can Dentists Work from Home?

Of course, working from home during COVID-19 was not welcomed by everyone. Working *from anywhere* was not a possibility for many dentists. In the first few months of the pandemic, dental practices were shut down alongside office buildings. "Stay at home" orders were in place. Travel was not permitted, nor was it safe. Even as the country began to open up, some dentists had to stay home to look after kids whose schools were closed or take care of family members with chronic conditions.

As businesses began to accept the "new normal" of working from home, many dentists felt stuck. Others saw an opportunity to change the world of dentistry. Interest in telehealth was already starting to rise before the pandemic, and dentistry was not excluded. We all know how much patients "hate the dentist." Would they hate it less if they could receive oral health care from the comfort of their own home?

Telehealth has benefits for both patients *and* dentists.

On the patient side, benefits include:

- Less time commuting to (or waiting at) the dentist's office

- Reduced costs

- Access to oral health care that would have otherwise been neglected

Dentists who are interested in remote work can see the immediate benefits of a rise in telehealth. Teledentistry will not replace the industry completely but will provide more opportunities for patients and dentists to interact with more comfort and convenience.

Some dentists have also found remote work in being an insurance claim consultant for companies like DentaQuest or Delta Dental. These positions help review insurance claims, fees, or codes in order to determine appropriate and accurate documentation and to prevent fraud.

In Chapter 8, I will also provide a list of non-clinical careers that allow you to use your DDS. A few of these careers come with the opportunity to work remotely. Do not reduce any "digital nomad" dreams that you might have to be just dreams. You can still work from home, work from the beach, or work from wherever you'd like while using your dental school degree.

Working Remotely

If you have the option to work from home full-time (or full-time for a few months of the year,) the future *could* look like working from "home" anywhere in the world. This was already the reality for many "digital nomads" and remote workers before COVID-19 hit. It could be a reality for you, too.

What Is a Digital Nomad?

"Digital nomad" and "location-independent" have both been terms used to describe a lifestyle of working remotely and traveling the world. Although the terms were first used in 2006, they didn't catch on until the 2010s. That is, before the global pandemic.

Digital nomad careers include:

- Programmers

- Web and app developers

- Graphic designers

- Writers

- Entrepreneurs

- Affiliate marketers

Before COVID-19 hit, searching for "digital nomads" on Instagram brought up pictures of laptops on remote beaches, Bali sunsets, and working out of a hammock. Blogs documented the experiences of digital nomads living in the farthest corners of the Earth. Groups like Hacker Paradise or Remote Year gave young people the chance to transition into the digital nomad life. For a fee, these groups would arrange accommodation, coworking spaces, and activities in up-and-coming cities, moving every month. All participants would need to do is have a remote job.

You do not *have* to sign up and pay a fee to become a digital nomad. If you want to travel the world and work remotely, all you need is a remote job and a little bit of direction.

If You're Working Around the World... Where Do You Work?

Digital nomads often travel to international hotspots for people living the same lifestyle.

These hotspots include:

- Bali, Indonesia
- Medellin, Colombia
- Chiang Mai, Thailand
- Buenos Aires, Argentina
- Lisbon, Portugal
- Budapest, Hungary
- Cape Town, South Africa
- Hoi An, Vietnam

What do all of these places have in common? They have a community, resources, and opportunities that are appealing to digital nomads. The right combination of the following features brings digital nomads over in droves:

Flexible visa options. If you want to extend your visa in Thailand or Indonesia, you most likely have to hop over to a neighboring country for a "visa run." Some countries offer visas specifically for digital nomads. Most digital nomads enter these countries on tourist visas, but easily find ways to stay long-term and avoid paying taxes.

Cheap rent. Would you rather spend $1,500 to rent an apartment in Austin, Texas, or $300 to rent an apartment in Buenos Aires? Rent prices in digital nomad hotspots are too tempting to turn down. Digital nomads may also choose to live in long-term hostels that cater to backpackers or location-independent people who don't mind living in a bunk bed.

Coworking spaces. For as little as $15 a night, guests at the Selena hostel in Medellin can enjoy a place to sleep, wake up to a continental breakfast in the morning, *and* access the hostel's coworking space. Coworking spaces have been surging in popularity. They're not just for entrepreneurs or companies of one. Digital nomads use subscriptions to coworking spaces to work anywhere in the world.

Coworking spaces don't just pop up in these hotspots, either. In 2017, there were 26,000 coworking spaces around the world. That number was expected to double by 2022, although COVID-19 may impact the construction and use of these spaces. Over 11,000 of these coworking spaces were in the Asia Pacific region, with almost 7,000 in the EMEA (Europe, Middle East, and Africa) region.

Communities of digital nomads. As I will point out later in this chapter, working remotely is not always as hip or exciting as it seems. Isolation and loneliness still exist among people who work from home *or* travel around the world. Without a sense of belonging, the mental toll of working in an office parallels the mental toll of working from home.

Fortunately, cities with large remote working populations offer opportunities to come together, mingle, and make friends. This sense of community exists in coworking spaces and hostels, but also exists in coffee shops and bars that cater to travelers. Language exchanges and other events allow people to meet locals *and* travelers alike. Couchsurfing, Facebook, and other websites are filled with these events.

The Future of Travel

The uncertain future surrounding the COVID-19 pandemic has many digital nomads "stuck" in their home country or the last place they traveled before the Coronavirus hit. Borders closed. Coworking spaces shut their doors. Language exchanges are harder than ever with masks or limited gatherings. Will it be safe, or even possible, to travel around the world?

Signs point to yes. As early as July 2020, countries started to *expand* their digital nomad visas, rather than shut their doors. Barbados and Bermuda began accepting applications for single people and families to work remotely in their countries for up to 12 months. Both countries reported fewer than 200 cases of COVID-19 when the applications opened. Although these countries were not considered "hotspots" for digital nomads in the past, a surge in tourism and a boost to local economies could give the countries the reputation and clout they need to attract coworking spaces and other opportunities for nomads.

Or Just Work from Home

The remote lifestyle is a popular dream among young people with no children, pets, or mortgages. Retired couples and families *can* live this lifestyle, but it is far from accessible to everyone. Location independence may become the "new normal" for many, but the digital nomad lifestyle will not.

You might have written it off immediately. You're not alone. The downsides to traveling the world full-time mimic the hesitations that many office workers have about working remotely full-time. Before you jump headfirst into negotiations or travel plans, take some time to weigh the common downsides of these lifestyle changes.

In fact, you may want to consider working remotely just so you can work from home. As changes in childcare occur, you might find you need to be at home more to take care of the kids. Having the ability to work remotely doesn't necessarily mean you have to travel, just that you have the freedom to work where ever you can. As dentists, you'll find that we are limited in this aspect. Our practice and our schedules often time don't allow us the flexibility to take our job home.

Inability to Collaborate and Communicate

The first drawback of remote work is the reason why employers hesitate to offer this option to their teams. According to the State of Remote Work Survey, the inability to collaborate and communicate remains the top struggle for remote workers.

This general frustration has a variety of causes: poor Internet connectivity, coworkers who don't know how to navigate *Zoom*, scheduling meetings, etc. Individuals may be able to tackle problems from the comfort of their own homes, but when they have to recruit coworkers, productivity could grind to a halt. This can be especially frustrating for anyone who is tasked with making split-second decisions. Questions can be quickly answered over the phone, but only if both parties are *next* to their phone. Sometimes, employees find it easier to pop into someone's office for a short brainstorming session or easy answer.

Every organization, healthcare or otherwise, has different problems daily and different requirements for collaboration. Some companies can easily communicate with customers online. Dentists can't offer most patients a solution unless the two are in the room together. Although the rise in remote work has led to innovations that improve collaboration between coworkers, there are still problems to solve and solutions to discover.

Dealing with Loneliness

The State of Remote Work Survey shined a great light on remote work. But although 99% of remote employees were happy to *stay* home, working from home is far from perfect. Researchers who study remote work seem to find the same problems popping up over and over again. One of these problems also exists within the dental industry: loneliness.

For dentists considering a career change, this problem is not new. As discussed in Chapter 1, dentists often feel lonely or isolated in their jobs. They may work alongside hygienists and see patients throughout the day, but without colleagues in a similar position, social connections may be strained.

Similar problems occur for remote employees. If the employee chooses to work from their home, they may only physically see one or two other adults throughout the workday. Coffee shops and coworking spaces allow remote employees to work around other people, but they are not always colleagues. (If two people in a similar job position *are* in the same space, they might not even know it.) Remote employees who want to vent about work or enjoy social interaction often have to wait for the clock to strike five. Office employees can just hop over to the next cubicle.

Digital nomads find themselves in similar situations. If they want to socialize with friends, they have to meet them first. This is a daunting task, especially in a country where you may be

128

unfamiliar with the language and culture. Companies like *Remote Year* are not just valuable because they arrange travel and accommodations. They also arrange friendships, social outings, and connections that may be obstacles for the independent traveler.

These are serious barriers to a healthy work-life balance and fulfilling life. Loneliness is more than just a feeling. It's an epidemic leading to the rise in health problems and premature mortality. Before these effects take hold, loneliness may just tip the scales of work-life balance.

Inability to Unplug

Without a distinct "office" and "home," many lines become blurry. Work is always just a few steps away. There are always more tasks to complete - and no physical distance stopping you from checking them off of your list. Coworkers and managers can reach you with a quick email or a text.

Inability to unplug followed loneliness on the list of struggles faced by remote workers. This may be a result of *where* employees choose to work. 80% of the remote employees who answered the State of Remote Work Survey said that "home" was their primary work location. Coffee shops, libraries, and other spaces paled in comparison.

The pressures described in Chapters 1 and 2 may follow remote workers if proper boundaries are not set. Data shows that we already have a tough time sticking to a 40-hour workweek if we are traveling to and from a physical location. When there is no commute stopping employees from working, how can they (or their managers) expect to stick to a strict 9-5 schedule? One benefit of a career in clinical dentistry is that a person is forced to practice only within the confines of the dental office during structured open hours.

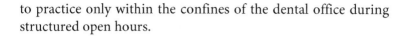

Blurred lines between work and home may also affect your physical ability to sleep at night.

In Chapter 3, I mentioned that 40% of Americans use their computers after 10 p.m. Some of those people are working, and not just from their home office. Data reveals that a *majority* of young professionals admit to working from their beds. This poses serious problems for young professionals who also want to get a good night's sleep. Sleep experts caution against working from bed, saying that bringing work to the bedroom prevents the space from being a relaxed, comforting environment.

If working from bed makes the bedroom a more frantic and stressful place, one might argue that general remote work does the same for the entire home. Unless work-life balance is a priority, remote employees could find themselves even *more* stressed out than when they were working in an office.

The Perfect Mix

There are obvious benefits to working from home that have not been listed in this chapter. Childcare, pet care, and the time you have to spend with your family drastically change when you are given the opportunity to work from home. Other drawbacks to working from home also exist. Working from home may come at a cost, both financial or in other areas of your life. The grass may appear greener on the other side. In reality, both "sides" have similar challenges that may affect your physical and mental health if they spin out of control.

Loneliness and the pressure to work overtime are not limited to an office or home environment. These problems, which contribute to an unhealthy work-life balance, can also be alleviated in the office or while working from home. The solution may not lie in *where* you work, but simply *how* you work. I used to be a provider who worked during lunch in an attempt to accommodate more patients. Boundary-setting is key to this solution.

The 2019 Udemy Workplace Boundaries Report revealed that changes within the workforce have encouraged boundary-crossing on many different levels. These boundaries may directly contribute to the common problems experienced by remote workers. There is the inability to unplug - 46% of employees feel pressured to work through lunch. Alongside the inability to collaborate is a confusion on *where* to collaborate with coworkers: 37% of employees believe that coworkers and managers are too informal on workplace chat or messaging. Feelings of loneliness in and out of the workplace may also *cause* boundary-crossings. More and more employees feel uncomfortable with coworkers bringing their personal life into the workplace. Those who are shut out from personal conversations may feel more isolated at work.

■■■I

The solution is to simply set boundaries in and outside of work.

■■■I

Be firm if coworkers are making you uncomfortable. Be clear about when you will be working and when you will be away from your devices. Once you have communicated your boundaries, stick to them.

Do not just set boundaries with colleagues. Set them with yourself. If you intend on getting a full eight hours of sleep, set boundaries. Put your digital devices away at a certain time and shut off your laptop. If you want to reduce the amount of stress that you endure at work, consider lightening your workload. Hold yourself accountable for uncovering and setting boundaries related to your schedule and salary terms.

There is no one solution to establishing a healthy work-life balance and enjoying your career. Explore the different opportunities that may become available and choose the options that work best for you. Use your upcoming career change, or even a return to the "old normal," as a way to reset and establish boundaries with your career as a dentist.

ACTIVITY: Find out how well you would work remote

√ Try out different areas and spaces like an office, co-op, or coffee shop.

√ Do you prefer to dress in business attire or regular clothes, how about pajamas?

√ What time do you feel most productive, in the morning or evenings?

√ What do lunchtimes look like? Will you eat out because you can or have everything you need at home.

√ Do you listen to music or prefer silence while working?

Re-Evaluating the Working World (and How It Affects Dentistry)

For some, the downsides of remote work are worth the price of flexibility, independence, and the opportunity to travel. For others, the downsides of the traditional 9-5 are worth the structure, routine, and balance that was previously established before COVID-19. If you are currently unsatisfied with your current job, changes might have to be made in the office or at home to spend your days without stress. One solution doesn't fit every professional. Everyone has different preferences, situations, and financial obligations pushing them one way or the other.

Even if you plan to stay in the healthcare field, it's important to know that the working world *is* changing. Dentistry, and other healthcare industries, is likely to change, too. Not all changes are going to be extreme. It's unlikely that every single one of your colleagues is going to pack their bags and move to Bali tomorrow. But there are plenty of compromises and smaller changes that could make a significant impact on where and when you arrive to work every day. The following policies and changes could be a staple of the post-COVID working world.

Part-Time Remote Work

Facebook and Twitter may be extending the option to work from home, but many companies are itching to get back to "normal." Working from home may just be something to ask for, rather than expect.

Remote work may also be something to *negotiate*. Employers may offer remote work one day a week, four months of the year, or another arrangement that works for both parties. This gives employees the opportunity to save money on childcare, live the digital nomad lifestyle "part-time," and enjoy a true balance between spending time at the office and spending time at home.

This would be an ideal scenario for someone looking to break away from clinical dentistry full-time but also keep up with their skill set by practicing a couple of days a week.

Shorter Work Weeks

Companies were toying with the idea of a shorter workweek *before* the COVID-19 pandemic. Study after study involving four-day workweeks suggested that the shortened schedule boosted productivity *and* saved money on resources. A Microsoft subsidiary in Japan shared that productivity increased by 40% after switching to a four-day workweek. After New Zealand firms started to implement four-day workweeks in their offices, Prime Minister Jacinda Ardern suggested that the country should adopt a similar policy. Ardern was less concerned with productivity and resources, and instead focused on considering a four-day workweek to encourage domestic travel.

Now that businesses have seen first-hand that flexibility in the workplace does not reduce productivity, *other* benefits of flexible hours are coming to light.

■■■

Remember in dentistry, more days worked does not equal more production made.

■■■

This is a flawed approach employers use to squeeze revenue out because of its simplicity. Do not be fooled! Take a look at your schedule and find reasons for productivity besides adding more workdays or hours

More Remote Employees Give Dentists More Flexibility

Dentists have faced more competition in recent years. This competition drives many private practices and corporations to extend their hours. Late-night and weekend hours give these practices a leg up on the competition by catering to the typical 9-5 employee. Of course, there is a trade-off; many dentists find themselves working these irregular hours *in addition to* the 9-5.

As more companies see the benefits of remote work and flexible schedules, there may be less of a need to keep doors open past 5 p.m. This isn't guaranteed, of course. But business leaders are no longer taking a "doom and gloom" approach to flexible workweeks. The benefits that arise from flexible schedules are still surprising business owners, employees, and the general public. If you are starting to realize that dentistry does not allow for the flexibility it once guaranteed, then a career change may be in your future.

Find Disruptions that Work for You

There will be drawbacks from the changes coming to the 9-5. Not every employee prefers working from home. Not every business leader has undergone a revelation about flexible working hours. The future is still unknown, both at the individual and company levels. As someone who may be contemplating a career change from dentistry, these are all important things to consider.

The future of the working world is changing for *everyone.* COVID-19, globalism, and trends in productivity have all introduced different arrangements for businesses and employees who are looking for a more satisfying work-life balance. A satisfying work-life balance looks different for everyone. The decisions you make about going back to work or pivoting your career may not look like your dental colleagues. But your colleague may also have a different living situation, financial situation, or preferences for working in the office.

Do not let uncertainty hold you back from planning your future. You can still negotiate your salary, go back to school, pivot your career, or start an entirely new venture during this time. The problems that you see may become a unique opportunity for disruption. Problems may also be an opportunity to wait out the storm and see how your business or industry changes for you. Be sure, however, to understand what changes you want to see, both in your work schedule *and* what pressure you take on every time you come to work.

At first, the world believed COVID-19 derailed the 9-5. As companies adjusted to the remote working world and overcame new problems, it appears that the 9-5 is just on a new course. This new course is moving faster into the future. Business leaders have confidence in a more remote workplace because they've lived through it.

■■■

Flexibility does not have to impede productivity.

■■■

With fewer people tied to strict hours and physical locations, *all* industries will have to adapt and seize new opportunities – including dentistry.

I know what you're thinking. All of this sounds great on paper: working by the beach, longer vacations, and a salary that supports your lifestyle and *doesn't* require you to work 50 hours a week. For many, the "future" of the 9 to 5 is a present reality. For others, this future feels out of reach. Dentists do not always feel "free" to explore careers outside of dentistry. This mindset, cultivated by generations of dentists and years of dental school, often leads new dentists to compare their industry with a cult. But as you will see later in this book, there are ways out.

Chapter 6:

The Cult of The Daily Grind

School typically doesn't prepare young people for life – unless their lives are spent following instructions and pleasing others. In my opinion, that's why so many students who succeed in school, fail in life.

– Ray Dalio

Former dentist – now successful career coach and founder of *Lolabees.com* – Dr. Laura Brenner, first described how dentistry is analogous to a cult in her blog post "Escaping the cult of Dentistry." Before I explain, accusing any group or organization of being a cult should not be done willy-nilly. When you think about the actual cults that exist in our world today, roping in dentistry seems like a far reach. In fact, most dentists only practice with one or two other professionals in their office! Cult members are surrounded by other cult members. They live with them, practice the same religion, and work toward a common goal together. But let's zoom out. Your office may not have a cult-like environment. The profession of dentistry as a whole, however, can be just as "hard" to escape. This holds many dentists back from making the career change that will provide a healthier work-life balance.

Cult leaders carefully demonize any opposition to the cult. Members who try to question the cult's rules or backstory are punished. Anyone who tries to leave is shamed and reminded of the "enemy" that awaits them at the door. Peer pressure is a powerful thing. It can make even the sanest people second-guess their knowledge and opinions. No one dental leader does this. Our society, however, has put dentists on a pedestal. That pedestal, aside from being lonely, may feel like a safe or powerful position. No one, including other dentists, their family, or just people they meet in passing, is likely to tell you to step down.

Dentists are in a unique position. They are *not* constantly surrounded by other dentists. Unless they attend conferences or continuing education, they might not see another dentist at all during their day to day. Up until 2005, the ADA reported two out of three working dentists owned a solo practice. No other dentists in sight. Half of all the dentists in the United States were the only person in their job position at work. Even associates only have one or two other dentists who can share responsibilities or discuss salary. Any concerns or complaints fell onto the ears of people outside the dental industry (if they were even expressed at all.) Let's be honest, how much can these people really understand terms and procedures?

Isolation has serious side effects. The isolation of dentists in private practices, however, have a unique consequence. There is very little community for dentists to express their grievances. Like a cult's efforts to silence a dissenter, individual dentists *also* remain silent about their pains. They feel as though they are alone in their struggles. No one is around that understands the physical and mental toll of dentistry. Without validation, a dentist may gaslight themselves or believe that they are the only one who is struggling in the industry. Hopefully you understand by now, that this is not true and there are many who have a similar outlook about dentistry.

When things are left unspoken, a person may be left even more confused about their position within an organization and the world. It is common for dentists to stay quiet and "soldier on" to not burden their family and friends with their frustrations. The fear of disappointing friends and family by leaving the dental industry is powerful, even if it is unfounded. The fear of judgment may override any desires to live, judgment-free, for yourself.

It's time to live for yourself. Education can be a powerful tool that allows you to break free from dentistry, cults or any organization that prevents you from enjoying a satisfying life. In this chapter, we will examine a handful of elements of indoctrination. These elements appear in all cults, inviting people to abandon their lives and become indoctrinated into the cult. All cults have a similar joining process: they catch people who are at a crossroads, make a soft sell to rope them in, and then begin to create a new reality for their new member. When a member decides that it's time to leave, they discover that this process is not so easy. The cult creates a fear of the outside world. They also use peer pressure from other members of the cult to keep members in.

These elements aren't just a part of cults but also pyramid schemes. One could also argue that you are "indoctrinated" into the dental profession. Not everything lines up, of course. The horror and violence within the most infamous cults are simply not present in the corporate dentistry or other businesses. But joining the world of dentistry (or many other professions today) offers similar promises to cults. And leaving feels just as threatening.

By understanding how we are roped into this "esteemed" profession, and forced to stay within, you can find an easier way out. I will end this chapter with the best strategies and tools for exiting a profession while still maintaining your relationships, freedom, and hope for the future.

What Is a "Cult?"

Despite sociology's success at "co-opting" the word cult in recent decades, cults are still generally used to describe religious organizations. Many of the most infamous cults in modern history have an element of religion to them.

Even with this new definition, cults are not your usual group. Political cults, therapy-based cults, and fitness-based cults exist in the thousands today. They often hold "socially deviant" beliefs, make fierce demands of their followers, and often resort to violence. Joining a cult always comes with grand promises and a better life. Leaving a cult often requires that you risk your life or livelihood, just to get your freedom back.

So why do we throw this term around? I'm certainly not the first person to compare the everyday working world to cult-like organizations. Along with Dr. Brenner, why does Forbes Magazine pose the question, "Are Successful Companies the New Cults?" Why does the Harvard Business Review ask, "Is Your Corporate Culture Cultish?" Why do friends and colleagues accuse co-workers of "drinking the Kool-Aid," a reference to the mass murder-suicide led by Jim Jones? (Many historians argue that his disciples actually poisoned themselves with Flavor-Aid, but let's not split hairs.)

One reason is that cults are just a part of pop culture. We are fascinated with cults. We devour documentaries like *Wild Wild Country*. There are groups of individuals who work the 9-5 and spend the rest of their time obsessing over Charles Manson. Even if you were horrified by the acts of the Church of Scientology, you might get a kick out of seeing their marketing materials in your mailbox.

Yes, there is something that draws us to cults. The elements that draw the individual into the cult are commonly the same elements that lead people to be fascinated with the idea of cults. Vox's *Cults Explained* says that "the eternal fascination

141

stems from the mystery of how their leaders exert such complete power." How did Charles Manson lead a group of teenagers to Spawn Ranch? Why did so many "normal" people abandon their lives to follow faith healer, Jim Jones? What does it take for someone to take out over $300,000 in loans, dedicate all of their free time to one cause, and put every priority at the bottom of their list?

Is that last question talking about a cult - or just becoming a dentist? Is the indoctrination process the same as paying a college hundreds of thousands of dollars, just to work at a job for decades to pay off your debt?

The Elements of Indoctrination

Not all of the elements of indoctrination are present in healthcare professions. In dentistry, we do not see one sole leader with the charisma and vision to convert thousands of people into cult followers. That isn't to say there aren't charismatic leaders in tech or other industries that resemble cults. Some charismatic leaders who adopt a following in non-religious industries have been known to appear in pyramid schemes or multilevel marketing organizations. These types of people are or organizations are very good at drawing you in and indoctrinating or "coaching" you to change your beliefs to accept the unreasonable or illogical.

Certain elements of indoctrination, however, are present in dental organizations:

- Members join when they are at a crossroads in their life.

- The "soft sell" of the dental field is hard to pass up.

- Once you dedicate yourself to becoming a dentist, you enter a "new reality."

- Leaving the dental industry means facing an "enemy" of the unknown.

- Dentists face peer pressure as they enter or leave the dental field.

Sign Me Up

People do not join cults because they want to join a cult. Cult-ish organizations provide promise. They sell a grand mission to help the world and change the fate of humanity. At the time, a person joining these groups believes that they are becoming part of something larger. They feel that this is the missing piece that will allow them to be fulfilled and complete. Everything will be okay, so it's worth it to sign their life and money away. A lot of professionals feel justified in putting their lives on hold for half a decade and being hundreds of thousands in debt to pursue this goal. In what other kinds of activity or instance does this make sense?

Crossroads

There is a specific group of people that join cults. They are often at a crossroads, looking for a change. Divorce, loss, and rejection send people into the arms of cult leaders who offer answers, solace, and a community working toward a common goal. Cults like the Rajneeshees or Peoples Temple formed in the 1970s. Young people at the time were living in a tumultuous era of American history. They wanted to see changes in the world and create a better life for themselves and their children. Joining the antiwar movement and the Civil Rights Movement allowed you to fight for a greater cause, but little progress appeared to be made. Cult leaders promised to save members and save all of humanity. This was very appealing, especially to people who had nowhere else to turn.

■■

People today who enter the dental field or working world face similar crossroads.

■■

They have to make a huge decision about their life. Parents, family members, and teachers are asking them where they are going to college. What are they going to school for? What profession will they enter once school is over?

Not all professions are treated equally in American society. Telling your family that you are studying to be a dentist garners a different reaction than telling your family that you are studying to be a plumber, a manager of a retail store, or an ad executive. Even if these 17 to 21 year-olds are aware that they need to take out loans, they are assured that they can pay them back later. With little financial education taught in today's high schools, students do not know any better. They don't know the costs of being an adult, of having a family, of paying back hundreds of thousands of dollars in student loans. Students entering high school do know, however, that dentistry is a respected and stable profession.

This is one of the reasons that children choose to enter the medical or business field. High school students rely on the knowledge of family, counselors, and (if you're lucky) mentors in their chosen field. They do not fully grasp the concept of the investment required to enter certain jobs, and what other responsibilities you will have to juggle as an adult. They are at a

144

crossroads, and the road that they follow is rarely chosen entirely by them.

The Soft Sell

The reality of a cult or pyramid scheme is never revealed until it is too late. Recruiters do not share the inner workings of these groups, the oppressive culture, or the strict rules. Instead, new members are shown the cult's supposed end goal. One group wants to help humanity. Another group wants to show their devotion to a certain idol. Yet another wants to help their members become their best selves. These great promises are a great motivator. The member's investment in these groups becomes a small price to pay for the larger reward in the end.

This reminds me of my early days of shadowing dentists. The promise of a career in dentistry was exciting. I observed dentists who had opened up a private practice months after completing dental school. The demand for dentists reduced the need for any marketing budget or advertising know-how. Three and a half days of working with patients was enough to make a living. The rest of the week was spent at home, with the family, or pursuing your passions.

Who cares if I was racking up a bit of debt? An extra few years of working four days a week was worth the flexibility and fulfillment that I would enjoy throughout the rest of my career. After all, the dentists I had shadowed were enjoying a debt-free life, right?

A career in dentistry used to be an easy sell. (Many say that it still is.) Family and friends will not discourage you from pursuing a career in the medical field. On top of the flexibility, high pay, and an enjoyable career, you are doing something that will make the people around you proud. The hours put into your

145

dental education are worth the knowledge and esteem that you will gain with your degree, right?

Creation of a New Reality

Once you commit to becoming a devoted member, it becomes your entire existence. Cult leaders control every move and decision that you make. Experts on cults believe that "mind control" is their greatest strength.

Within mind control, cults exercise different types of:

- Behavior control
- Information control
- Thought control
- Emotional control

How you feel, where you go, and what you do are all controlled by the cult. You start to lose sight of the life you had before the cult. Leaders encourage members to question their family and friends, abandoning them if they go against the teachings of the cult. Members of many cults are called to abandon all of their belongings or even their clothes. The cult gives them new clothing, names, living arrangements, and job assignments. A member's identity is completely erased and replaced with one that lives and breathes for the cult. Every moment of their *life* is influenced by the cult.

Although I have kept the same name since I entered dental school, I have added a D.D.S to the end of it. Although dentistry may not be as extreme as a traditional cult, it can harbor some of the same emotional responses. The process of creating a new reality begins before you even enter the working world. By the time you have finished dental school, you are prepared for this new reality and assimilate easily.

Dental School

Any student studying dentistry will tell you that the workload is anything but easy. It's not uncommon to spend over 40 hours every week on schoolwork. Classes, studying, labs, exam prep, and extracurricular activities related to dentistry fill up your schedule quickly. Students who must work while in dental school find little time for sleep, much less any other social activity. Hobbies, passions, and recreation are pushed to the side so the student can achieve a larger goal: to earn their degree. Many dental students who are attending school while supporting their family or raising children must make sacrifices in order to successfully graduate.

Extreme Workload

The degree is in your pocket. What's next? A similar schedule. Instead of schoolwork, new dentists are consumed with "real world" work. For some dentists, "real world" work consists of opening up a new practice: ordering machinery, teaching yourself how to handle business operations, and establishing yourself in the area where you set up shop.

Other dentists find themselves consumed by the culture of corporate dentistry.

The glory days of dentistry are over. The "soft sell" I mentioned earlier does not apply to today's dentist. Why? First, student loans get in the way. It is hard for anyone to carry the burden of $300,000 in debt and work three days a week.

Second, dentists worked three to four days a week because *they* wanted to work three to four days a week. They made their own schedule because they were in charge of making their schedules. If you work for a larger corporation, that power is taken away from you. Dentists face more pressure to work longer hours. In some cases, they have no choice. DSOs or demanding private practice owners may offer little to no paid time off or vacation days. They have an assembly line of patients ready for a dentist to see morning, noon, and night. Leaders at the top are less concerned with the schedule and quality of care of each individual dentist, and more concerned with their bottom line. If that means keeping a practice open on weekends to accommodate patients, so be it. If that means staying open at night, so be it.

Leaving the "Cult"

When new graduates are looking for work, they may check sites like Indeed or Glassdoor. These sites contain reviews of different corporate dental practices that scoop up a lot of new graduates after they get their diploma. From personal experience, I was strongly encouraged to write a review immediately after I started working before I had time to assess the company culture! There are reviews that praise these companies, while reviews from actual *dentists* aren't so easy to find. Account managers, receptionists, and HR managers can all leave reviews on each individual company.

There are a lot of common themes in these reviews: there is little work-life balance, low pay regardless of job position, and managers have little experience in the dental field, not enough support, or budget issues. If you look at company culture, one word comes up again and again in positive reviews: family. Employees are treated like family. This message is spread throughout the company to boost morale and create a sense of unity within the company. A family atmosphere is known to be a loving atmosphere - but is that even true for all families?

When a corporation "becomes" your family, your other family has to compete for time. When a cult becomes your family, you're well on your way to indoctrination. Accepting this organization as a family is a tactic for bringing people into a cult *and* keeping them there. After all, people do not abandon their families!

Introduction to the Enemy

Cults have strategies that prevent people from leaving. They introduce the idea of an enemy, often woven into the story that the cult paints when members are joining. Members of a cult may be positioned as a "chosen" few. These few people will survive after the fall of mankind, an apocalypse, or the second coming. Everyone else (including people who have left the cult) will be attacked, sent to live in eternal damnation, or simply wiped off the face of the Earth.

If you truly believe in the stories told by a cult, leaving sounds like a death sentence.

Leaving dentistry is not so dramatic. No one is going to be attacked for trading in their dental drills for a certification in personal training. Any dentist who has voiced concerns about their future in the field knows that there are consequences to leaving.

The same praise that friends and family give to new dental grads may turn into questions and judgments when the grad wants to go back to school. Spouses, despite seeing the stress that the dental industry puts on individuals, may be concerned for their finances. There is a certain status that one enjoys when they are in the medical profession. Is someone really willing to give that all up, just so they can see reduced hours at work?

The "enemy" of the dental profession is the alternative career to the dental industry. Dentists cannot easily transition into other jobs. Management positions and entrepreneurs do not need four years of education regarding molars and canines. Even if a dentist has another job position or industry in mind, there are questions as to whether their skills are transferable to get them a job.

If a dentist *doesn't* have a plan, the "enemy" can be the unknown. In Chapter 10, I outline ways that you can prepare and *plan* for your next adventure in life. Without a plan, it is likely that you will waste time and money investing in a career that may not suit you. Knowledge is power. Once you develop a plan for your career change, you can exercise your power and break through the pressures of leaving the dental industry.

Leaving Dental for Other "Cults"

When you plan your switch, consider that dentistry is not the sole industry facing accusations of being "cult-like." Corporations that have never touched a tooth may have a more cult-like culture than your average DSO. Be aware of this trend - it can save you from leaving one cult and jumping into the arms of another one.

Built to Last is one of the best-selling business books out there. It influenced a whole generation of managers and business leaders. In the book, the authors compare the Walt Disney Company to a cult-like culture. It's not a bad thing, either:

"Architects of visionary companies don't just trust in good intentions or 'values statements;' they build cult-like cultures around their core ideologies."

In the eyes of a business leader, being compared to a cult might not be so damning. A leader can thrive by creating an environment in which employees sacrifice their time and money to belong to their company. Working overtime, forgoing vacation, and accepting lower wages puts more money in the pockets of the people at the top. If you can create a cult-like culture, other leaders may consider you to be a visionary, too.

Leaving dentistry does not mean you are free from all professions or companies that function like cults. Disney, Walmart, Soulcycle - these are all successful companies, and they have all been accused of having a cult-like company culture (or one that extends to their customers.) Be vigilant of the industry and the companies that you may choose instead of dentistry. Remember, you are at a crossroads. You are undoubtedly looking for change and acceptance in a new career. This is the time when cults swoop in and do their best work. Do not fall victim to spending tons of money on multi-level marketing and dental practice building courses on the hopes that these programs will make you feel passionate about dentistry again.

151

Do not forget what your original purpose and goals are in determining your career change.

So, You Want to Leave... Now What?

The thought of leaving dentistry (or any profession) does not last a day. You may experience months or years of swearing that you are going to quit within the month, only to stay put. Do not let insecurities, the unknown, or pressure from others hold you back. If you are thinking about leaving dentistry, consider making small moves (and keeping yourself in check.)

ACTIVITY: Which small goals have you started to implement in initiating a career change.

— Update Resume

— Discuss ambitions with friends, family, and colleagues

— Write down passions and transferable skills

— Create a list of potential careers

— Search Job Listings

— Consult with Career Counselor/ Mentor

— Take courses in areas that interest you

— Create a financial safety plan

The Importance of Seeking Out Support

What moves should you make to help you through this transition? For the answer, we look to a pyramid.

In the 1940s, psychologist Abraham Maslow set out to outline how humans prioritize their needs and create a fulfilling life. He created a pyramid-shaped structure called *The Hierarchy of Needs.* Within this structure are humans' most basic needs (food, water, and shelter,) and the ones that we seek to fulfill only after all other needs are met (self-actualization.)

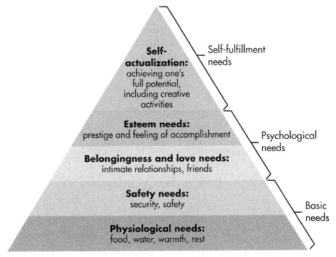

Image obtained from simplypsychology.com

Somewhere in the middle lies love and belonging. People want to feel as though they are a part of something bigger. This is why many people join a cult or choose a career in the dental field. A membership in an organization or a job title becomes *proof* of that belonging. One of the perks of joining the dental field is telling people that you are a dentist. You immediately belong to a larger organization of medical professionals with a niche specialty and power. When you contemplate leaving the medical field altogether, you contemplate removing yourself from this group in which you belong to something larger.

This lack of belonging keeps many people in cults, jobs, and industries for decades. Never mind that a job pays the bills and fulfills the physiological needs at the bottom of Maslow's pyramid. Jobs like dentistry can fulfill your needs all the way up to the top of the pyramid, even if the costs of fulfilling those needs leaves you wanting more.

So, what do you do? Find replacements. Replace your job with another source of income (or savings) that fulfills your physiological needs of shelter, food, and financial security. Seek out support, no matter where you are in your career. If you are new to the dental field, experiencing burnout, questioning your job satisfaction, or taking the plunge, seek out support.

Above love and belonging are greater needs: esteem, feelings of accomplishment, respect, and self-actualization. It is much harder to achieve these larger goals if you do not have a supportive group where you truly belong. Take this time to seek out support and find a community that will help you move through this new phase of your life.

■■■

You are not the first person to feel trapped in the "cult" of dentistry.

■■■

The right mentor or buddy can see where you are coming from and give you advice based on how *they* exited a job that wasn't right for them.

How to Connect with Dentists

Validation from peers will help you move forward, *and* it is easier to access than you might think. Sure, there might not be other dentists in your office. You might not have "dentist friends." There are still ways to reach out to fellow dentists and seek guidance about your possible career shift.

Surprisingly, Facebook comes in handy here. There truly is a Facebook group for everything: "Helping Dentists," "Desi Dentists in the USA," and "Pediatric Dental Forum" are just a few of the Facebook groups catering to dentists. Groups for dentists in specific cities can also narrow down your group. (There is even a group for "Dentists who ride...a Pelaton!" if you need that kind of specific support.) Social media groups offer a way to connect with other dentists who may be experiencing the same frustrations as you.

Facebook groups and other forums can also help you:

- Find jobs and partners in the dental industry

- Give and receive solutions to specific problems that might make your job a pain

- Bounce around other ideas related and unrelated to dentistry

- Let off some steam!

You may not need to leave the dental industry entirely. Sometimes, you just want to be heard by someone who understands you. Take advantage of these groups, even if you intend to be a dentist until the day you retire. We all need a sense of community to reduce stress, seek out support, and feel like we belong.

Do Not Forget a Supportive Community Outside of Dentistry

A Facebook group of dentists is unlikely to follow you into your next journey. In addition to seeking support from people in the dentistry field, seek out support from people who *aren't* in the dentistry field. This might be as easy as reaching out to your friends and family.

■■■

Be honest about your struggles.

■■■

Share your concerns about the physical and mental tolls of the profession. Friends and family may not know what it is like to be a dentist, but they will not understand your frustrations until you voice them. A supportive group of friends or family will listen, even if they are worried about the "enemy" outside of the dental industry.

I was lucky to have friends from college who didn't eat, breathe, and sleep dentistry. They were fellow advertising majors. Although they can't tell a ceramic crown from a zirconia crown, they know how to listen to a friend who is struggling. Stepping away from the pressures of dentistry was easier when I had this group of friends by my side. Evaluating my career has also reminded me how much I value a group of friends.

The Greater Good

At the end of her TED talk speech, "Why Do People Join Cults, educator Janja Lalich says, "Believing in something should not come at the cost of your family and friends, and if someone tells you to sacrifice your relationships or morality for the greater good, they're most likely exploiting you for their own."

As you start to examine your current job position and companies that you would like to join in the future, keep these words in mind. You should not have to sacrifice time with your family or your friends just to get a steady paycheck.

Part III
Plan to Pivot

Chapter 7:

Finding Balance

(Outside of Clinic)

Life is like riding a bicycle. To keep your balance, you must keep moving.

– Albert Einstein

COVID-19 has completely shaken up the country's economy and the "typical" work-life balance of a dentist, healthcare provider, or other employees. Now is the time to evaluate your work-life balance pre-COVID. Were you satisfied with the amount of time you spent at the office and at home? If not, what can you do to balance the scales and start getting more satisfaction out of life?

No two dentists will have the same answer. Factors like family, finances, and current work-life balance will also impact how satisfied each dentist feels (and what it will take for them to live their most fulfilling life.) Some dentists will decide that the best way to achieve work-life balance is to step away from their current position and find a job that brings them more joy. Another option is to work as a dentist part-time and pursue other passions or jobs part-time. A third dentist may need to renegotiate contract terms and adjust their schedule to feel more

160

satisfied at work. The right work-life balance may be achieved as a dentist *only* after setting boundaries and adjusting your schedule. I cannot tell you what is best for you, your family, and your financial situation. Only *you* can determine that for yourself. Only *you* can take the necessary steps to reach your goals. I merely want to help you realize if you even need or want to make a career change in the first place.

This chapter will explore basic strategies and tactics that you should follow whether you choose to walk away from dentistry, stay in the industry, or pursue other passions. The right choice will make itself apparent to you as you continue to understand your priorities and what brings you satisfaction.

Leaving Dentistry Completely

You feel unfulfilled. You're stressed and your health is at risk. Long hours at work prevent you from enjoying life and seeing your family. After weighing all of your options, you believe that it's time to walk away from good. If work is disrupting your work-life balance, stepping into a less demanding field can adjust the scales.

Walking away from a job is not easy. The pressures from family, friends, and colleagues described in the last chapter are just the tip of the iceberg of emotions that come with swinging into a new career. Of course, you are not the only person to walk away from their job. The Bureau of Labor Statistics reports that the average person holds *12* different jobs throughout their lifetime.

Once you have made the decision to leave dentistry, embrace the change. Do not look back. A new career or venture may feel like a journey into the unknown, but this leaves room to be pleasantly surprised. Switching jobs may encourage you to discover a new passion or deepen your relationships with family and friends. Your newfound freedom may bring new friends into your life, or give you the opportunity to expand your family. In one, two, or five years, you may look back on your life and be thankful that you left your career.

Do not let your *entire* journey be a surprise. Just like *you* have a vision for your future, your friends and family do, too. Take time as you transition to communicate, explore, and plan for this new chapter in your life. With the right planning, you will be able to discover yourself, your relationship with your family, and what you truly want out of a "job" or "career."

Discovering Yourself Again

"When one door closes, another door opens." You have probably heard this phrase time and time again. As you step away from your job and "close the door" on clinical dentistry, remember that the "door that opens" might not look exactly the same. The opportunities available after leaving the clinic may not be a dental job or even one in the healthcare field.

As you transition from the world of dentistry to a new career, you have the opportunity to discover who you are. In the first chapter of this book, I mentioned how dental school (and a dental career) can envelop your entire life for years.

You lose sight of who you are, because you spend all of your time thinking about dentistry.

162

If you step away from dentistry, you'll have a lot of time to think and explore with your personality, passions, and dreams.

ACTIVITY: Write down a list of your interests. I'm not just talking about subjects that you currently explore in your everyday life. Think about activities, talents, and hobbies that you are interested in trying for the first time. When you have a healthier work-life balance, you can actually take time to explore these interests.

MY LIST OF INTERESTS

1. _____   5. _____

2. _____   6. _____

3. _____   7. _____

4. _____   8. _____

Discovering Your Family Again

Remember, you are not the first person who has questioned their career or made big changes to feel more fulfilled in life. Do not go through this journey alone. A supportive community of family, friends, and colleagues can help you through this transition. People who have gone through similar journeys can help you along the way. You can help people, too. Alleviating the demands from clinical dentistry allows you to give back more to the community that is supporting you. Through this process, you will be learning more about yourself as an individual. You will also be learning a lot about the people who mean the most to you in your life.

As you contemplate your decision, take time to sit down with your partner or family. Have a family meeting or take a weekend trip. Find some time where you can really sit down, put away distractions, and talk about your job transition and what that means for your family unit. Don't be afraid to ask big questions. What role have you taken on in your relationship or family? What are your family's expectations as you transition into a new career? Do you have expectations for your family as you start on this new journey? How will finances and family budget look?

There are many jobs and responsibilities that come with taking care of a household and being a parent. Chauffeuring children, managing property, and attending to basic chores all come with the role of "partner," "parent," or "homeowner." As you transition out of your career, you may be expected to take on some of these jobs. Be prepared to have this discussion and balance your new responsibilities at home.

These new responsibilities and role expectations come with great rewards. Driving your kids to school in the morning gives you extra time with them. Working around the home gives you a greater appreciation for the work that you have done to build your life. Fewer distractions from work allow you to be more present for the people that matter most. Your family may face struggles as you transition into a new job, but these struggles are no match for the bond you will form and time spent together.

Discovering What It Means to "Have a Job"

The role that your job plays in your life will look very different than the role that dentistry once played. (Isn't the whole point of leaving dentistry to gain a healthier work-life balance and work a less stressful job?) By leaving your job, you have an exciting opportunity. You have the chance to control what role a job plays in your life. You have the ability to determine how much you will invest in a career, both during this transition and over the next few years.

Dentists spend years in school *just* to get a job. We endure the physical and mental toll of *just* to keep their job. This investment is not unique to dentistry, but it's certainly not a common practice across all industries. It takes between six months and two years of training to become a police officer. Real estate agents need to complete 180 hours of education before they can go out into the field. Day traders, investors, and entrepreneurs just need knowledge of the current market to start earning money and cutting their workload in half. Other jobs don't require employers to hold certifications. Employees just need to show up at the office every day to make an income. Jobs like affiliate marketing require you to set up systems and build a following initially so you can continue to earn passive income while you sleep.

If you earn passive income, your "job" may be nothing more than a way to fund your lifestyle. This sounds like a dream to some, but a nightmare to others. Careers play a different role in the lives of different people. You may want more or less out of your job than your partner or neighbor, and that is okay. Again, this transition into a new career allows you to define what needs your job fulfills.

Jobs can be more than just a source of income. They can:

- Help you establish a routine
- Allow you to feel that you belong to a larger group
- Challenge you physically and mentally (in a healthy way)
- Build up your self-esteem
- Connect you with people around the world
- Help you help people in your community and beyond

What do you want out of your job? These are the questions that you should be asking yourself, not only as you pivot to a new career, but also if you are sticking with your career in dentistry. Dentistry can fulfill some of the roles listed above. Dentistry can also do the exact opposite. Adjusting your schedule, employer or career can be the key to working in a job that fills the roles that you envision for your career.

Boundaries and Scheduling

As you explore other opportunities, you might see that dentistry *does* meet your needs. With a few adjustments, your career can be a satisfying source of income without being a position that overtakes your life. You might come to this conclusion, or you might not. If you *do* decide to stick with your current career, evaluate how and where you can make a change. No one "magically" achieves a healthy work-life balance, especially in a demanding career like dentistry. Take action toward creating a healthier work-life balance. You may feel uncomfortable taking this action, but stay strong. The discomfort of adjusting your schedule or setting boundaries is worth the satisfaction and healthy work-life balance that will result from your efforts.

Schedule Vacation Time

If you are keeping your current job, do not disregard the advice regarding self-discovery and communication with the people closest to you. A change in your work-life balance will likely affect your availability at home and relationship with your family. Check in with your spouse, children, or friends about how your career affects your relationship. Hear what advice they have for you, and what responsibilities they want you to take on as you make changes.

Want to feed two birds with one hand? Schedule a vacation. Try to save or budget appropriately and spend time off of your phone to completely focused on your family. De-stress and reconnect with your loved ones, even if that means disconnecting from work. Using vacation days (and not responding to work calls during your vacation) is the first step in setting boundaries at work and establishing a schedule that works for you.

Re-evaluate Your Social Media Feed

Remind yourself through this process that *you* are different from other dentists. You might have different responsibilities, skills, patients, and obligations. The reasons *you* might want to stay in dentistry or leave the industry may vary from the dentists that you know, and that's okay.

How do you keep in touch with other dentists? Usually, it's through social media. This creates a paradox, as social media is listed by experts as one of the biggest contributors to the "loneliness epidemic." Social media, in the dental industry, may also be a tool to compare ourselves to other dentists. The rise in "Instagram dentistry" has led to a surge in feelings of jealousy and insecurity for dentists who may not have (or can perform) what they see on their feeds. But even the "best" dental social media influencers do not tell the whole story about a practice, patient, or clinician. Do not let photos or a quick caption add more stress to your life. If you are sticking with the dental industry, you are probably facing enough stress as it is.

As you create boundaries with your employer, create boundaries with yourself. Does social media (dentistry-related accounts or otherwise) make you feel insecure? Do you spend more time scrolling than you would like?

■■■

Try not to give too much weight to what other dentists showcase and focus on your own goals and skills.

■■■

Refraining from social media will not give you a raise or create more hours in the day, but this small step could have a big impact on the way that you see yourself in the world of dentistry.

Get Rid of Distractions

One of the easiest ways to cut your ties with social media is to evaluate its purpose in your life. Social media has some legitimate purposes: you can connect with people or learn something new by scrolling through your feed. If you don't have an intentional purpose for scrolling, you are using it as a distraction.

Eliminating distractions from your life can help you get more satisfaction out of *everything* that you do. Distractions prevent you from seeing your true potential. You are reading this book because you want to use your full potential. As you begin to take this journey, keep an eye out for distractions, and replace them with actionable steps that will help you reach your goals.

Remind Yourself of Why You're in the Dental Field

The road to a healthier work-life balance is not just in cutting the amount of time you spend at work or on social media. Find ways to *value* the time you do spend at the office more. Maybe that value comes from standing your ground against corporate leaders who are not trained in dentistry. Or that value comes from being able to focus and carefully examine each patient without the clock ticking or serious stress. One quick and free way to add more value to your time at work is to practice gratitude.

You chose the dental industry for a reason. Salary, freedom, and the opportunity to help others may be the fuel that keeps you going, even when times are tough. Remind yourself of the things that brought you to this field (and keep you in it.) One way to practice gratitude is to keep a "gratitude journal" in the mornings. Before you drive to work (or as soon as you get into the office,) write down 3-5 things that you are grateful for that day. This daily habit can give you a little mood boost, even when your schedule is stressful and things are going awry.

ACTIVITY: Jot down at least 5 things you really enjoy about your current position as a dentist. Don't write down what you think you should enjoy about being a dentist, only the things that are present in your current job. If you can't get to 5 easily, that may be a sign it's time to re-evaluate your situation.

TOP 5 THINGS I REALLY ENJOY ABOUT MY
CURRENT JOB:

1. _____

2. _____

3. _____

4. _____

5. _____

Hold Yourself Accountable

In Chapter 1, I listed a series of actions that you could take to alleviate the mental and financial stress that comes with a career in dentistry. These actions include (but are not limited to):

- Refinancing your loans or adjusting your budget

- Evaluating (and changing) how much time you spend on hobbies

- Setting boundaries and expectations to lighten patient load

- Researching and implementing salary negotiation tips or practice management protocols

- Seeking out a professional therapist

All of these actions can lead to a healthier work-life balance. I bring these actions up again because these are not one-off actions. Each of these tasks may require a regular commitment, follow-ups, or reinforcement. Setting boundaries, for example, requires sticking to those boundaries and communicating if they have been crossed.

Before you set these plans into motion, consider how you will hold yourself accountable. How will you ensure that you have stuck to your budget, or explored new hobbies, in a month from now? Two months? One year? If you don't hold yourself accountable for the changes you want to make in your life, you can easily slip back into your old routine (and unhealthy work-life balance.)

Reach out to someone who can be an "accountability buddy." Accountability buddies can be a spouse, a friend, or a colleague in the dental field. Share your goals and ask them to hold you accountable every few weeks or months. You can do the same for them. Even better if you know another dentist who is looking to make a similar career change! Check in regularly about what actions you have taken to secure a healthier work-life balance and make your career more enjoyable. Accountability buddies add an extra element of motivation and push to help you take proper action at work or home.

Setting boundaries and holding yourself accountable are key components to reaching your goals, whether or not you want to stay in dentistry, walk away entirely, or find a happy medium between the two. Discipline will carry you a lot farther than motivation.

Pursuing Your Passion

If you're currently considering a career change, then chances are you probably don't consider dentistry your "passion." Do not worry - you don't have a lot of catching up to do. Only 13% of Americans feel passionate about their job. Deloitte Insights states that more than two-thirds report that they are simply not engaged with their work. Americans that *are* prioritizing their passion are making an interesting discovery: not everyone *has* a passion. The discussion around "following your passion," much like the discussion around remote work, has changed over the last few years. If you feel that you have been missing out on pursuing a passion, take a listen into what experts are now saying about how this fits into your general career.

Develop a Passion Before You Follow It

What *is* your passion? Is this a question that you feel prepared to answer?

Again, do not feel as though you have a lot of catching up to do. In 2018, researchers Carol Dweck, Paul A. O'Keefe, and Gregory M. Walton dissected the term "follow your passion."

There are some surprisingly problematic implications of this phrase.

- The phrase assumes that each person has one passion.

- The phrase also assumes that your passion is "fixed" and that every person has one passion that is "set" from the time they are born.

- Once you have "discovered" your passion, you must follow it. Following it implies, to some, that you should abandon other interests.

This idea of a "fixed" passion parallels a "fixed" mindset. Dweck, author of *Mindset: The New Psychology for Success,* argues against the idea of a "fixed" mindset. She suggests that by adopting a "growth" mindset, one can manifest growth in skills and traits that they want to pursue.

Research from Dweck, O'Keefe, and Walton make similar suggestions about passion. Passion, they believe, is not "fixed." The phrases "follow your passion" or "find your passion" only set people up for disappointment. Instead, the researchers suggest that people *develop* their passion.

Consider this phrase as you explore what will play into your work-life balance. You do not have to immediately jump into one specific area of interest. If you are not seeing immediate "results" from your hobbies and interests, do not consider this time to be wasted. Focus on how you feel while trying new things, not what achievements you can get out of developing a passion.

Your Passion May Not Be a Source of Income... At First

"Achievements" include money. Dentistry is not the only field that puts pressure on people to perform. Everyone, to some degree, feels the pressure to produce something that they can share with others. Young people often feel trapped by this pressure as they pursue creative projects and passions. Will this passion get them "likes" on social media? Will they be able to turn this passion into a "side hustle" or even a six-figure income?

173

Remember the intentions behind picking up a hobby or pursuing a passion. If you feel the pressure of turning a hobby into a side hustle, you will not change anything about your work-life balance. "Perfection stress" will simply change hands from dentistry to your new hobby (or continue to pile up until it consumes your work *and* life.)

Following Your Passion? Try Recognizing Your Strengths

Earlier, I mentioned that the phrase "find your passion" can set people up for disappointment. Why? People assume that their passion automatically falls in line with their strengths and skills. They get excited to follow the passion of their choice, feeling accomplished after making basic strides. But the research from Stanford University finds that people who have early success "following their passion" are most likely to abandon it later. The researchers observed participants who believed they had one single interest and those who were more open to exploring interests in different areas: STEM, arts, etc.

Participants with a single interest were more likely to believe that their skills and strengths fell in line with their passion. Indulging in their passion was easy. As the participants progressed, they found themselves hitting a stopping point.

To someone with a "fixed mindset," or the belief in a single "fixed" passion, this stopping point was a sign to give up. These participants believed that they reached their limits. If they were not going to get any better, what was the point of pursuing their passion further?

Researchers supporting the idea of a "growth mindset" or "developing your passion" see this stopping point as just another obstacle. If you want to build on *any* skill or area of interest, you are going to encounter problems or challenges.

Advocates for a "growth mindset" are more likely to face these challenges head-on, overcome them, and continue on their journey.

Consider if you have a "fixed mindset" or a growth mindset" towards dentistry.

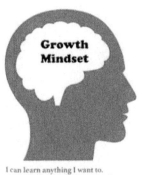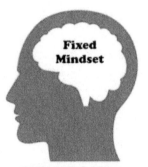

	Growth Mindset	Fixed Mindset

I can learn anything I want to.
When I'm frustrated, I persevere.
I want to challenge myself.
When I fail, I learn.
Tell me I try hard.
If you succeed, I'm inspired.
My effort and attitude determine everything.

I'm either good at it, or I'm not.
When I'm frustrated, I give up.
I don't like to be challenged.
When I fail, I'm no good.
Tell me I'm smart.
If you succeed, I feel threatened.
My abilities determine everything.

Created by: Reid Wilson @wayfaringpath ⓒⓉⓈⓄ Icon from: thenounproject.com

FIXED MINDSET		GROWTH MINDSET
• SOMETHING YOU'RE BORN WITH • FIXED	SKILLS	• COME FROM HARD WORK • CAN ALWAYS IMPROVE
• SOMETHING TO AVOID • COULD REVEAL LACK OF SKILL • TEND TO GIVE UP EASILY	CHALLENGES	• SHOULD BE EMBRACED • AN OPPORTUNITY TO GROW • MORE PERSISTANT
• UNNECESSARY • SOMETHING YOU DO WHEN YOU ARE NOT GOOD ENOUGH	EFFORT	• ESSENTIAL • A PATH TO MASTERY
• GET DEFENSIVE • TAKE IT PERSONAL	FEEDBACK	• USEFUL • SOMETHING TO LEARN FROM • IDENTIFY AREAS TO IMPROVE
• BLAME OTHERS • GET DISCOURAGED	SETBACKS	• USE AS A WAKE-UP CALL TO WORK HARDER NEXT TIME

If you *are* interested in one particular passion, keep these conclusions in mind. Do not give up. Do not let roadblocks or obstacles hold you back from doing what you want to do. At first, following a "passion" might feel easy. Nothing is ever easy if you want to continue to develop your skills.

How to Develop Your Passion Without Failing

If you "follow" a single passion, you may find yourself repeating history. You invest and invest in your passion, with little return (sounds a little like the journey of becoming a dentist). Instead, experts suggest that a healthy alternative to following your passions is recognizing your strengths. As you recognize your strengths, you can find ways to contribute that are fulfilling, successful, and don't require the investment of developing *other* strengths.

> Try to find yourself using your strengths in ways that align with your passions.

Here's an example of how identifying strengths *and* aligning them with your passions can bring you fulfillment. Say you have a passion for fitness. You love fitness and make a priority of going to the gym in the mornings. In your ideal world, you spend every day in the gym, sharing this love with other people. If you could go back and do it all again, you might have chosen a career as a personal trainer.

But your ideal life comes with costs. In your area, you find that personal training is not as lucrative as you would like. You don't want to go through the certification process, only to face a lot of competition. After discussing your interests with mentors in the field, you realize that the pay cut and lack of job security might not be worth the career switch. There are also elements to the job, like being in the spotlight, that you feel are out of your comfort zone.

Instead, to balance out your stressful career, you identify your strengths. You have a knack for writing and always have.

Writing is just one of your many strengths, but it is one that you can pursue from anywhere. Similar to fitness, you do not see the benefits of dropping your dental career to pursue writing. As long as you have a prompt or a story to tell, you can take your mind off of the stresses that come with your "day job." In this example we see that although fitness can be a passion, writing is a strength that could be leveraged to blend the two together into a productive venture.

For me, I realized that although I wasn't necessarily passionate about dentistry, I did consider it a strength. I was very knowledgeable about my field and was technically a very proficient clinician. What I *was* passionate about, was writing and helping others figure out their goals and purpose. That is when I decided to combine the two into the product you hold in your hands now: this book.

There are numerous ways that you can blend your strengths and your passion. In your spare time, you can spend little to no money and start a blog. On your blog, you write about fitness, try out new products, and share your secrets. You could even cater your blog to dentists and other healthcare professionals who are looking to combat the physical tolls of dentistry. The blog is a hobby, but one that you just enjoy as you unwind at night.

Another way to blend your passion and strengths is through grant writing. Grant writers help corporations, nonprofits, and charities apply for grants. After just one course, you can apply your skills as a writer to this niche. You work with charities that help to bring fitness classes and education to underserved communities. Grant writing can even become a lucrative career.

These two examples are very different, but find a way to blend a strength with a passion. Writing and fitness seem to be unrelated at first glance, but with a little creativity, you can bring them together (and even make some cash on the side!) As you explore your passions, strengths, and priorities, you might find the right hobbies or side hustles that bring you joy outside of work.

How to Identify Your Strengths and Passions

People typically do not discover their strengths or passions overnight. They need years of failure, success, and experimentation to truly identify what makes them unique. If you can't immediately pick out a strength or passion to combine, do not worry. Remember, it's never too late to discover new things about yourself.

The following resources *can* help you get started on the path toward recognizing your strengths and passions:

- Enneagram Personality Test
- Big Five Personality Test
- Meyers-Briggs Personality Assessment
- Career Aptitude Tests

These tests can offer some insight into your personality and the "roles" you have created for yourself. They are not a substitute for going out, trying new things, and exploring what you like to do. Be patient, be open-minded, and do not think too hard about what you would like to try. If you are interested in learning something new, go for it!

Chapter 8:

Creating Solutions

Every system is perfectly designed to give the results it gets.
– Paul Batalden

In the previous sections of this book, you have been able to take a peek into what dentists (and other professionals around the country) are experiencing. You know that the bright smiles that dentists show off on social media may be hiding stress, pressure, and the financial burden of student loans. As DSOs and dental franchises continue expand and set expectations for new clinicians, the weight of this stress is only going to increase.

The grass isn't just greener outside of dentistry - it is actually a whole meadow of opportunity. You have many options for stepping out of the dental industry and into a profession that allows you to develop your passions and have a healthier work-life balance. If you want to pivot to a new profession, you can. If you want to improve the role that your current job plays in your life, you can. All it takes is some planning, patience, and (most importantly) action. This section will allow you to explore *all* of those options, including some options to take action and stay in your current job position.

We have reached the part of the book where we must talk about taking action. Action may look like negotiating for a higher salary, creating firm boundaries with your employer, or searching for a more fulfilling job. This action may take days, weeks, or years. Some of these actions will be more challenging than others. As we will explore in this chapter, the right mindset and perspective will allow you to take these actions *and* feel confident that you are on the right path toward a more fulfilling career.

The right mindset is built around one idea: jobs are created to find solutions to problems. On this journey of changing careers or re-evaluating your job, you too must find solutions. The first three parts of this book have addressed the problems that current dentists face in their job. Finding the right solution will not only solve those problems - they will improve your life.

"Finding solutions" does not encompass all of the effort and time that you will need to get the job done. But these two words can help you put your past choices, present situation, and future actions into perspective. When you chose to enter dental school, opened a private practice, sold the practice to a DSO, or took a break from work, you were looking for solutions. You can continue to look for solutions as you enter this new phase of your life.

Choosing a Career Too Early

Many people stay in a job that they don't love because re-evaluating your career and passions as an adult feels strange or wrong. If someone, at the age of 30, 40, or 50, tells you that they are looking to take a career aptitude test, your first instinct may be to question them. Career aptitude tests are traditionally given to high school students who barely know themselves. The suggestions within these tests are meant to be an answer, or at least a guide, for a child with their whole life ahead of them.

Let's take a step back. How much sense does this process *really* make? We expect young adults, at 17 or 18 years of age, to make a choice that will impact the rest of their life. With barely any "real world" experience, this person must choose the role that they want to play for 20, 30, or 40 years. Seven years before a child's brain fully develops, high school students are pressured into choosing a college or career. Due to the current costs of a college education, this decision comes with a burden of $30,000, $50,000, or $100,000 in debt. Before the age of 30, this young adult must carry that burden and start working.

You may have chosen the dental field at 17, 18, or in your early 20s. Do not look at this decision as one to regret. You knew you had a long road ahead of you, and that your education would be more rigorous than most. Not only did you stick to your education when things got tough, but you also graduated and obtained a license from the state dental board.

■■■

Look at your education as proof that you can choose and succeed in another career.

■■■

If you can pass dental school, you can pivot into any career of your choice. The hardest part of making a shift is finding out which direction you want to take. Once you have figured out your next moves, you can put *half* the amount of time and energy into it as you did dental school. Success will follow.

Throughout this book, you have learned the effects that an unfulfilling and stressful job can have on your mental and physical well-being. Now, it's time to look at jobs that will provide you with a flexible schedule and the chance to develop your passions and purpose. This chapter takes a closer look at alternatives to a dental career and how to find a job that satisfies you. Do not let a choice that you made in your early 20s determine the course of your life. Do not sacrifice your mental and physical well-being for a career that is not fulfilling you. Take a deeper look into what you want to accomplish and what careers will help you.

What Problems Do You Want to Solve?

Jobs play a specific role in a person's life. In the previous chapter, I listed some of the roles that jobs can fulfill. Your place of employment may provide you with a sense of purpose, connect you with like-minded people, or simply provide a source of income that is needed to fulfill your lifestyle.

If you are looking for a *new* job, zoom out. Think not only about the roles that jobs fulfill in *your* life but also how jobs solve problems in a larger society. The right people in the right jobs solve problems. If you want to find the right job for you, you might want to first find the problems that you want to solve.

Dentistry Solves Problems... But Comes with Other Benefits, Too

People need dentists. Unfortunately, there is no vaccine for tooth decay, gingivitis or the pulpal necrosis. The U.S. needs dentists to perform upwards of 15 million root canals each year. Dentists do solve problems that will continue to occur as long as people have teeth.

Did you enter the dental industry to solve these problems? Not everyone does. A career in dentistry provides (or previously provided) a long list of benefits that exceed the desire to perform a gum graft. The American Dental Education Association has a list of why people choose to be dentists.

This list includes:

- Independence and a flexible lifestyle
- A high salary
- Being a respectable member of the community
- Providing care to the community
- Working as part of a team

Does the list above align with the list you made in the previous chapter's activity of things you enjoy about your current situation as a dentist? Or is your job missing some or many of these elements dentists find appealing in their profession?

This list is extremely appealing. No wonder dentistry is becoming a more competitive industry! As many dentists have discovered over the years, this list also creates a Catch-22. The benefits of a dental career attract many dentists to the field and to open their own private practices across the country. More dentists drive competition. More competition requires dentists to work longer hours, put more money into operating costs, and search harder for patients to serve.

As you evaluate your career and your priorities, ask yourself: are you getting the benefits of the dental career that you were promised when you entered dental school? If not, what options do you have (in and out of the dental industry) to obtain those benefits in your job or your life?

■■

For each problem that you want to solve, you can find
dozens of jobs that work toward a solution.

■■■

This is true in the dental industry, too! Although 80% of
dental school graduates choose to open their own private
practice, professionals who are passionate about oral health can
use their degrees in different job positions. You can indirectly fix
smiles and make a difference in one of these non-clinical jobs.
For some, getting out of direct-patient clinical care might be the
key to staying in dentistry.

Academia or Research

The stress and competition within the dental industry is
not stopping students from pursuing dentistry as a career.
Predoctoral enrollment is at its *highest* level in history. Over
25,000 students enrolled in predoctoral dental programs. (This
number is up significantly from the early 1980s when dental
school enrollment experienced its last "peak." In the 1980-81
school year, just under 23,000 students were enrolled in
predoctoral dental programs.) The ADA reported eight schools
throughout the country received their initial accreditation and
welcomed new students over the past 10 years. New dental
schools are continuing to open up and are expanding the overall
class size by increasing enrollment. Dental schools will need to
increase the professors and faculty members to keep up.

Dental schools need professors to usher in the new
generation of dentists, but professors need more than just a
degree in dentistry. Academia and research reflect the working
world, and professionals who can adapt to remote learning and

online instruction are more valuable than ever. This could be the perfect position for younger dentists who are burnt out by working with patients but still want to contribute to improving oral health.

Dental professors are also able to focus on any areas of research that could advance the field. If you have interest or experience in the laboratory and enjoy experimentation and writing grants, then turning to academia and research dentistry might be just the solution.

Be aware that you may need a masters or Ph.D. before you can become a dental school professor. The switch to academia may require extra years of schooling but will allow you to elevate the way that dental treatments are performed without directly working with patients.

Dental Malpractice Lawyer

From dentistry to...law school? It's possible! Malpractice suits are on the rise. Dentists (and patients) want to hire a lawyer who has knowledge of the dental industry. The combination of a DDS and a JD is a powerful one. If you want to continue making a high salary and flexing your knowledge of dentistry, becoming a dental malpractice lawyer may be the right move for you.

Of course, one of the biggest drawbacks of this choice is the costs that come with law school. Earning your JD may require three to five years. Your DDS will work to your advantage, but it will not replace certain requirements to *get into* law school. Start studying now.

Positions Within Dental Organizations

Education does not end when you get your degree. Dental school graduates may also find themselves working in positions handling continuing education and accreditation programs. These positions help organizations uphold the integrity of the dental profession.

Scoring a position in one of these organizations may not be as easy (or as lucrative) as a general dentist gig. This job could require years of networking, attending conferences, and fulfilling other duties outside of your private practice.

Do not let this dissuade you from looking for jobs outside of your practice. In the final chapter of this book, I will lay out the best practices for switching jobs and finally working in the position that you want. This could take years of saving, planning, or waiting for the right job to open. If you are interested in a non-clinical job that requires a dental degree, start looking *now*.

Dental Products Industry

Corporate dental practices do not just employ dentists or professionals in the oral health field. Experts in marketing, business, and finance also contribute to these practices. A successful DSO blends a clinician's expertise in dentistry with a manager's expertise in running a business. As you have learned through your work in the field or by reading this book, the blend of dental and marketing expertise is not always successful. But the combination of dentistry and marketing does not just exist within DSOs. If you are looking to work outside of private practice, you may want to consider a career within the dental products industry.

The jobs in the dental products industry range from "consultant" to "executive." Companies like Procter and Gamble (manufacturers of *Crest* and *Oral-B*) prefer professionals with dental experience to take these roles, even if your responsibilities do not include using products on patients.

There are advantages and disadvantages to careers in the dental products industry, too. The job may require an MBA or a background in marketing in order to successfully perform all of the responsibilities set by the company. Large dental products companies may have headquarters in a different part of the country, requiring you and your family to uproot your life and move somewhere new.

Keep an open mind when looking at non-clinical jobs, but remember what role you want a job to serve in your life. Jumping from one job to the next will only be successful if your new job improves your work-life balance, reduces stress, or offers more fulfillment.

Insurance Claims Consultant

Product developers are not the only professionals that need a dentist's expertise. Insurance companies may also look to dentists to evaluate claims. Working as an insurance claims consultant can be a sweet deal for former dentists who want a flexible, remote position. You can review claims from your living room, send them back, and get a heap of cash in return. If you want to choose this route, start networking now. Like an executive position within a DSO or dental association, you will need to know the right people to be considered for a job as an insurance claims consultant. These jobs are in demand. Spots are filled before you can say "bicuspid."

Military Dentistry

After weighing the pros and cons of these pivots, you might discover that you want to hold a clinical job after all. You still have options for adjusting your schedule, seeking out a different type of employer, and directly solving oral health problems by treating patients. One of these options is to serve as a dentist for the U.S. military.

Dentists are eligible for direct appointment to the Navy, Army, and Air Force after a thorough background check and screenings. Once enlisted, dentists may be required to complete physical training and military policy and procedure. This could be an ideal position for dentists who are looking to sell their private practice - the Army allows dentists up to the age of 60 to sign a two-year contract and start practicing. (Age limits for the Navy and Air Force are 41 and 48, respectively.)

Enlisting in the military, entering into the world of academia, and applying for a position within a larger organization takes time. You may need to develop skills outside of the ones that you employ on a daily basis. No career change is easy or stress-free. I list these non-clinical jobs as a reminder that you can find a solution to the mental and physical toll of your current job while staying in the oral health field.

Downside to Dental Career Alternatives

The above careers are not an exhaustive list of dental career alternatives, however, it's important that whatever interests you, is able to provide you with the aspects of dentistry you previously felt passionate about. It's important to note that if having an extremely high earning potential is critical for you, then some dental career alternatives will leave you discontented. However, if dentistry is ultimately what you enjoy, then maybe the money doesn't matter. Dental career alternatives also tend to be harder to break into and typically require a personal recommendation from someone currently in that position, more education, or the need for relocation. Make sure you find someone that may be in these fields of interest to help you better make the decision to pursue a non-clinical dental career.

Things Change, Including Your Passions

At 18 (or 28), you might have approached dentistry with gusto. Fixing someone's smile brought you great satisfaction. Running a private practice might have been your end goal when you entered school. At the heart of these goals is the passion to provide care, specifically oral healthcare, to others. Oral health is a very niche problem to solve. Maybe you entered dental school with the desire to help patients solve their oral health problems. If you still feel the passion for these problems and finding oral health solutions, the job positions I just listed could be the pivot you need to live a more fulfilling life.

Maybe you *don't* feel a passion for providing oral health solutions anymore. That's okay. Do not let your past goals, or your past accomplishments, hang over you. Plans change. Ambitions change. Priorities change. Parenthood, changes to an industry, and other factors can rightfully influence the problems that you want to solve and the demands that you have for your career. Instead of reflecting on what you wanted in the past, think about what you want *now*. Take the time to develop your passions. Remember, passion is not "fixed." My colleagues and I may have spent the past few years developing our passion for dentistry, but at some point, we all came to the realization that we did not want to develop our passion further. You have the option of developing a new passion or exploring solutions that have nothing to do with oral health.

The World Has Changed

Why is it so important to focus on the present moment? The world has changed immensely over the past one, five, 10, and 20 years. Opportunities are available now that may not have been possible at the beginning of your career or education. Problems that need solutions may not have been apparent. Instead of focusing on what choices you could have made *before*, focus on what solutions you can look for *now*.

Take the tech industry. My colleagues and I have been blown away by the advances made in technology since we entered dental school. At the time, the tech industry was in its infancy. YouTube was a place for people to post "random" videos. Facebook was for college students. No one predicted that it would shape advertising, marketing, and communication. "Social media" was not a popular term in the early 2000s. Now, students can choose to pursue a *Master's Degree* in social media marketing or management.

Facebook was not initially built to make tens of billions of dollars in revenue. No one went to college ten years ago to become a "digital nomad." If you told someone 20 years ago that you wanted to study the programming coding language, Python, they would ask why you were so interested in working with reptiles.

Careers in the tech industry are rapidly growing each day and the need for programmers, coders, and developers are in high demand. Most of these positions may not even require a degree if you have experience and most of the training you can receive can be inexpensive or free to learn on-line. The University of Texas at Austin offers a 24-week coding bootcamp that will train you in a multitude of coding languages while you maintain your working schedule. Companies like the *Salesforce* offer free and complete training modules to use their software. Acquiring this low cost or free education can be used to open up new doors in achieving a position in a tech company. Obtaining an expensive and time-consuming bachelor's degree may no longer be as useful as it once was.

If I could step into a time machine with the knowledge that I have now, I would have chosen to forgo my advertising degree and dental school education for a career in coding or development. My colleagues have expressed similar feelings. You, too, might have made different choices with the knowledge that you have now. But you, my colleagues, and I do not have a time machine. No one could have planned for the impact that the tech industry would have on the job market. No one could have planned for the impact that a global pandemic would have on the country in 2020. All of us were asked to make a decision at a very young age with the same level of uncertainty. We still do not know what the world will look like in 10, 20 years, or what jobs will be the most lucrative. You cannot plan for what the future will have in store for you, the job market, and the country as a whole. What you *can* do is look at the problems of today that you can solve in the future. Don't let the next 10 to 20 years pass by and regret not making the career change that could positively impact not only you but the world.

What Problems Do You Want to Solve?

The world has changed. Society has solved many problems and created many *more* problems. Each of these problems calls for an idea, a strategy, or a person with the responsibility to create a solution. When you discover the problems you want to solve, the jobs and tasks ahead of you become much more clear.

Here is an exercise to help you brainstorm the problems *you* can solve. Before you decide to abandon dentistry

191

completely, assess the problems that you want to solve in this world.

ACTIVITY: Physically write down some of the problems you see. Get creative! Think on a local, national, and global level. How are people struggling? What policies, procedures, and products need improvement? What information, products, or skills do people need in order to live their most fulfilling life?

PROBLEMS THAT NEED A SOLUTION

1. _____

2. _____

3. _____

4. _____

5. _____

Take a look at the company *Udacity*. They realized that obtaining a degree from a public four-year college costs an average of about $23,890 in tuition and is continuing to rise (outpacing inflation). The founders understood this problem and created a solution for the rising education costs and a progressively competitive job market. That's when they developed the "nanodegree." *Udacity* is an online education service, charging students a small monthly fee for self-paced programs that teach everything from software programming to artificial intelligence. By solving this industry problem, Udacity has risen to be $1 billion valuated company.

This list could take *years* to write. Do not try and write down every single problem facing the world today. Use this simply as an exercise to get creative and see how many opportunities you have in your career. People have problems that dentists can fix. But they also have problems more suitable for programmers, real estate agents, or entrepreneurs.

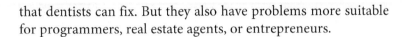

The greatest minds have been able to solve problems that people didn't even know they *had.*

If you chose to go to dental school in order to fix smiles and provide oral healthcare, you might still find fulfillment in the dental field. If you are among the people who prioritize flexibility, providing care to the community, or a high salary, it may be time to reassess why you are in your career. There is a job that can solve all of the individual problems that you can think of. Some of these jobs *also* offer a flexible schedule, an avenue to help the community, and the other benefits that many people seek out when entering dental school.

Reassessing your career and purpose may not be the easiest pills to swallow; during this process, do not judge yourself. Young adults (or children) make decisions to pursue a career. Ten years down the line, they may be happy with their career choice. They may also decide to switch careers, as many people do.

Really, Get Creative!

When I tell you to get creative with this list, I mean it. Think about problems taking place in your backyard, literally *and* figuratively. Brainstorm all of the problems you face (or improvements that you can make) as you drive to work, drop your kids off at school, or start your day. Write down problems that can be solved overnight. Write down problems that require centuries of research, work, and collaboration. Could this list point you to your new career? Possibly. Could this list also point you toward a hobby or passion that you can develop outside of work? Absolutely! Pivoting your career, as I will describe in Chapter 10, takes time. Spontaneously quitting your job today will not set you up for a fulfilling career tomorrow. In the meantime, you can find smaller problems.

Examples of these smaller problems may include:

- Teachers at your child's school don't have proper supplies for the year.

- Your yard is overgrown.

- A friend on social media is having trouble finding a job.

- Store-bought gifts for friends and family aren't cutting it anymore - they need something more personal.

- The kayak in your garage has not seen the sun for years!

- Your dental colleagues who have begun to feel unfulfilled in their career (wink wink).

All of these smaller problems have solutions that could turn into hobbies, passions, or even jobs. Look at these problems with your friend. With a little creativity, you can come up with solutions to help you and your friend. You could:

- Spend some quality time with your friend and help them de-stress.

- Share this book with your friend (and others) and form a book club.

- Browse for jobs that might fit your friend's interest (and do some research for yourself, too)

- Hold a networking lunch with your friends and colleagues who may be able to connect your friend with professionals in their field.

All of these actions can help your friend solve their problem. These solutions can also turn into something larger. Your networking lunch could become a monthly occurrence. As you plan these networking lunches, you develop a passion for connecting people or hosting events. If you can get the events sponsored or create a membership program for your events, you may even be able to turn one small problem into a lucrative side hustle. Or, it remains a hobby that allows you to feel accomplished and get your mind off of the stress at work. Your "day job" is stressful, but you can find joy in what you do outside of work.

If you don't look forward to work in the morning, you can at least find something to look forward to throughout the day. Finding the solution to a problem is not only rewarding, but it also helps to make your world a better place.

This is Not an Overnight Process

Burnout doesn't happen overnight. Neither does recovery. If you want to solve problems with a hobby, a part-time job, or a full-time job, you will need to plan properly and be patient.

Think about the time that it took to finish dental school, open a practice, and reach the point where you are today. The day you decided to enter dental school took place years before you started practicing. Even if you are one of the younger dentists that experienced burnout within a year of entering the "real world," you did not get to where you are now overnight.

Think about this when you are making plans or just making a list of problems that you would like to solve. Small-scale problems can become great hobbies. Large-scale problems can become lifelong passions or even careers. The solutions you create to both small-scale or large-scale problems can both fit into your life alongside your job. Give yourself time to grow, explore, and tinker with these solutions as you transition out of your career. The first solution to every problem is not going to be ideal. You may need to go back to the drawing board a few times before you find a solution that works without causing additional problems.

Let's go back to the example about the networking lunch. The first event attracts a few people but leaves you wanting more. What can make this lunch better for everyone who attends? The next month, you tailor the lunch to a specific industry. Attendance improves, but you find yourself spending too much time advertising the event. The next month, you charge a small fee to cover the costs of advertising, but you charge too high. After the fourth or fifth lunch, you find a budget and process that satisfies everyone involved *and* doesn't overwhelm you. In five months, you have found a solution that could turn into a business venture. But you needed to develop your passion, try out new things, and be patient before this could happen.

Transferable Skills

Transferable skills are any abilities you possess that are valuable in other careers or other employers in different industries or fields. These could include skills like dependability, organization, teamwork, or other assets employers look for in applicants. The transferable skills acquired from becoming a dentist can be applied to careers outside of dentistry when presented in the right way.

For example, communication is an important skill that employers look for in any candidate applying. If you have the ability to convey important and detailed information to patients or staff in an effective way then you can probably apply them in any workplace. Perhaps you are great at time management due to handling a full schedule of new patients while performing treatments efficiently. Maybe you are excellent at leadership and teamwork because you have trained your front desk and assistants into being successful and productive. You could be proficient in data analysis due to your ability to analyze periodontal charting in order to develop a diagnosis based on clinical attachment loss.

ACTIVITY: Circle some potentially transferable skills you've obtained in dentistry hat could be applied to any workplace.

Teamwork	Technology	Time
Leadership	Literacy	Management
Dependability	Flexibility	Multitasking
Communication	Problem	Creativity
Organization	Solving	Critical Thinking
Adaptability	Data Analysis	

The Right Mindset Will Keep You Moving Forward

The focus of this chapter has been on identifying problems. However, don't forget that the title is "finding solutions." The beginning of this book has also identified problems, both in the expectations placed on employees and the physical and mental toll of dentistry. As this book shifts to

197

information on changing careers, our mindset must shift as well. You have identified some of the problems that you are experiencing at work. You know that you are not alone. Other dentists also experience the physical, mental, and emotional toll of this stressful job. Now, it's time to find solutions.

As you explore your passions and hobbies, look for solutions. As you evaluate the ways in which your job is leaving you emotionally drained, look for solutions. This mindset will help you move forward even when problems continue to arise or change takes longer than you had anticipated.

■■

No matter what life throws at you, you can
(and will) find a solution.

■■

In the next two chapters, I will provide *some* of the solutions that can help you leave your job for good and plan for a successful career switch. These solutions may not be ideal for your financial situation, family structure, or location. Do not be discouraged if the solutions I provide are not perfect. The advice in Chapters 9 and 10 can be a good place to start brainstorming your *own* solutions. Dentists working for one DSO may find more success with salary negotiations than dentists working for another DSO. Parents may find that switching jobs may increase childcare costs *or* that the right job can alleviate those expenses.

Take time to evaluate solutions and how they might fit into your life. Be patient, be positive, and continue to move forward with the mindset that you are *finding solutions*. Your career should solve problems, not create a slew of new ones that rest on your shoulders. If you do find yourself facing more problems and unable to come up with an effective solution, it might be time to walk away entirely.

Chapter 9:

Leaving Dentistry

"Fun is one of the most important – and underrated – ingredients in any successful venture. If you're not having fun, then it's probably time to call it quits and try something else."

– Richard Branson

Dental support organizations come to dental professionals with a "solution" to their problems. They offer to employ associate dentists or even buy out an existing practice to handle the operations and marketing side of business. All a dentist has to do is what they do best: treatments, exams, and other dental procedures.

Dentists have learned the hard way, that this "solution" may create more problems. They are tied to corporations or smaller multi-office franchises that put their bottom line above the patient and employee welfare. Corporate or franchise dentistry is often run by people who have not completed a day of dental school in their life. The only "problem" they face is how to make a higher profit. If the solution is reducing staff or not updating equipment, they will choose that solution without much consultation from clinicians.

If you work for a practice you don't own, you could walk out and be replaced before the month is over. Dentists who opted not to own practice are waiting in line for a job and a salary that can help them scrape by as they pay their student loans.

You know the mental and physical toll that dentists are undertaking in order to stay employed full-time in their industry. If you find yourself in a similar situation, know that it is time to look for a solution. The stress, exhaustion, and unhealthy work-life balance that employers put on dentists are not worth holding onto a position that can be filled in a week's time.

It's time to look for a solution. Staying in your position, but negotiating your terms to fit a five-year plan and promote a healthy work-life balance, may be the best solution. Scaling back at work and setting boundaries may be the best solution. Walking away entirely may be the best solution. Not all of these plans can be executed tomorrow. Once you decide on the path that you want to follow, use the information in Chapter 10 to help you create a plan.

How to Stay and Negotiate Your Terms

When dental students shadowed professionals working in the "Golden Age of Dentistry," they saw dentists who worked on their own terms. These dentists had the freedom to open a practice, set their own schedules, and perform the procedures they enjoyed. The dentist who opened their practice was able to practice the way they wanted without insurance dictating treatment, without expensive marketing, or lots of debt. Dental students dreamed of the days where they could call the shots at work and make a lot of money doing (while providing quality patient-focused care, of course).

Dentists who are not satisfied with their position in a DSO or as an associate dentist may look back to these days with envy. Previous generations of dentists, while not completely free from stress, had enough control in their practice to recover and reduce stress when things got out of hand. Do not let these memories of "the good old days" take you down a path that will cause even *more* stress.

If you have been reading this book and relating to the mental and physical toll of dentistry, do not buy or start your own dental practice. Buying or starting your own practice to stay in your career is like having a child to save your marriage - you are only creating more complications when you do decide you have to leave. The costs of buying or starting a practice will only add a heavier financial burden onto your shoulders. Freedom is not as exciting when you feel trapped into working more hours and accepting more patients just to pay off the opportunity to have more freedom.

Instead of buying your own practice, look at the job you are currently holding. Can you stick with your current job and be satisfied with different terms? If the answer is yes, make a plan. Assess what salary will make you happy or what terms will allow you to work with less stress.

Assess Your Ideal Salary

A boost in salary may be the answer to your frustrations at work. Tight budgets can hold your family back from expanding or hold your partner back from quitting *their* job. More money can also help you pay off your student loans faster, or save up for a vacation. If you plan to retire early, you have to make more money now. In our society, more money means fewer limits.

Evaluating your budget is one of the first solutions that I provided for alleviating the stress and pressure that you might be facing. If you want to ask for a raise, take things one step further. Determine your ideal budget. Right now, you may be denying yourself trips to the chiropractor or vacations because you want to pay off your loans or put money into your savings account. Consider those expenses in a more comfortable budget.

As you write up your ideal budget, include the following monthly expenses:

- Rent, mortgage payments, and other living expenses
- Other bills (phone, Internet, etc.)
- Insurance
- Student loan payments, or other types of debt repayment
- Other monthly spending
- Retirement contributions
- Other savings

Add all of these expenses up. This is your pre-tax total. Add 20% to this pre-tax total, and multiply the answer by 12. The result is your ideal salary.

This number might be far off from what you are making right now. Do not be alarmed. Consider the change in expenses from when you began your career as a dentist to now. If you received a pay cut during your career or did not receive consistent raises, your pay likely hasn't caught up with the rate of inflation. Now is the time to "play catch-up." This number is a great starting point, or goal, for negotiations.

Look at the Terms of Your Contract

Happy with your salary, but not with the "perks" of your job? Negotiate the terms of your employment. Ideal conditions will vary for every dentist. A dentist who is expecting their first child may negotiate for different terms than a dentist who is newly single and wants to travel. Look at your priorities and the big picture and put together a list of demands for yourself. Some examples include:

- Associate responsibilities
- Work hours and schedule
- Potential Buy-out or buy-in of a practice
- Guarantee Rate or Per-day minimum pay
- Retirement contributions
- Healthcare benefits
- Tuition reimbursement

Also, discuss other areas specific to your position at your practice that could help ease the load a little offer and offer you some peace.

ACTIVITY: Check off items that you could consider reasons for you to stay with your practice or with clinical dentistry in general.

— Remove certain staff members or assistants that make your life hell.

— Maybe hire additional staffing or assistants

— Newer equipment or special instruments and supplies that could make treatment easier

— Reduce or change hours seeing patients

— Ability to refer treatments you feel uncomfortable performing

Again, you do not have to ask for a raise in salary to reduce the mental and physical toll of your job. Adjusting your work schedule or receiving parental leave may be the solution to your largest sources of stress. Find the terms that work for *you*.

Know what you want before you step into your employer's office. Most likely, you will have to negotiate. Be prepared for some back-and-forth before you and your employer settle on changes that will satisfy both parties.

Negotiating Best Practices

Once you have gathered your ideal demands, take these steps:

> **Gather a list of your accomplishments and contributions.** Employers do not care that you need a raise to alleviate stress or pay off your student loans faster. They want to know why you *deserve* a raise. How can this renegotiation benefit *them*?

Accomplishments may vary:

- Awards or recognition for your work
- Bringing referrals or patients from your former practice to your employer
- Consistent 5-star reviews on Yelp or other sites
- Loyalty to the company for several years

- Advanced CE training or certifications you've acquired

Consider the costs of paying you, and how you have managed to justify these costs throughout your career. Dental employers are *investing* in you.

What have you provided in return?

Research current trends and norms. Between 2013 and 2018, Forbes reported the average dentist's salary rose 6.8%. In 2019 alone, the average salary increased by 3.2%. Did your salary increase that much? Have statistics like this on hand when asking for different terms. Find out if costs of treatments have risen over the years or if the average percentage of collections has increased for providers over the years. If other dentists in your industry are seeing pay increases, why shouldn't you?

Keep in mind the costs of hiring a new employee, too. Employers need to spend thousands of dollars to hire someone new. Does your employer want to spend extra money hiring someone with less experience, or is it in *their* best interest to throw you extra vacation days each year instead?

Prepare what you want to say. Research and planning are key to a successful conversation with your employer. You will most likely be met with hesitation and you *will* be questioned by your employer. If your employer wants you to elaborate on *why* you deserve a raise, have something prepared. Roleplay this conversation with your partner, a friend, or a career coach if you want to practice.

Ask for more. Hiring dental practices are looking to reduce their overhead and budget in an attempt to increase profits. They will counter whatever offer you make and try to meet you somewhere in the middle. So, go high. If you are looking for a 2% raise in production pay, ask for 4%. If you want 14 additional paid vacation days, ask for 21. If you were to ask for 14, your employer would likely try and negotiate down to 7. Go high. In the best-case scenario, you get a better deal than you had hoped. Most likely, you will end up with terms closer to what you want.

Use silence. If your employer comes back with an offer, do not speak immediately. Silence makes people uncomfortable. Take a few deep breaths as you assess the offer, prepare your next thought, and make your employer sweat. After 15 seconds, they may feel uncomfortable enough to break the silence and give you more. Your employer may also know this trick, and use it against you. Be comfortable pausing and thinking before you speak.

Offer your employer time to think about your conversation. Employers will feel more comfortable if they feel the ball is in their court. They may also feel that their hands are tied, and need to seek approval from upper management before they can give you the terms that you want. If you are not happy with the direction of your negotiation, ask your employer if they would like a few days to think about what you want. (Of course, if you get an offer that satisfies you, go ahead and come to an agreement in your meeting.)

You have called this meeting because you are not happy with the salary or terms of employment that you have right now. If your employer refuses to budge or does not want to accept your accomplishments and value, consider your next steps. Start planning a pivot. Look for other positions with better terms or start saving to go part-time. However, you may want to leave the dental industry entirely. Weigh your options, but do not rely on a company that would rather replace you than meet you where you are.

Scale Back

If you are employed by a DSO, some terms may be relatively out of your control. Ultimately, your employer determines how much you get paid, how many vacation days are on the company's dime, and the healthcare plans that you and your family will be offered. If you are running your own practice, or feel trapped by your company, it might be time to scale back.

In the beginning of this book, I mentioned that I was on track to leave the dental industry entirely. I must admit that for a number of years, I have been working part-time. Years ago, I entered the industry because I was passionate about dentistry. Then, dentistry took over my entire life.

■■■

I could not be passionate about a career that was causing more stress than fulfillment.

■■■

After making a plan to enter a new career, I scaled back to working two days a week. (I will talk more about this plan in the next chapter.) This transition allowed me to see dentistry as a *hobby I enjoyed,* rather than a career. Since I've scaled back to working two days a week, I have fallen in love with dentistry once again. The money I make while working as a clinician is simply a bonus. Dedicating more time to other passions has allowed me to practice with a renewed focus and enjoyment. Scaling back, or working part-time, could be the right path for you, too.

How to Begin Scaling Back

Reducing the number of patients that you see can help to reduce some of the day-to-day stress that comes with working as a dentist. A less stressful job gives you more opportunities to think clearly, be productive, and feel joy, rather than dread when you walk into the office.

The financial pressures of attending dental school encourage many dentists to treat everyone that comes into the office and do every procedure that they need. Treating every patient that walks in and filling your schedule past your limits may increase your salary, but also increases the risk of:

- Working overtime
- Rushing to get to the next patient
- Making a mistake
- Treating a grumpy patient who leaves a bad review
- Getting hit with a malpractice suit
- Dental board investigations

When the "best-case scenario" is working overtime, it's time to take a step back. "Scaling back" looks different for every dentist:

- Refer out patients that make you uncomfortable or stress you out

- Reduce the treatments you perform to avoid high-anxiety cases

- Limit your hours and days at work

- Reduce the number of new patients you take on and focus on existing patients and continuing treatment

208

If you continue to make a habit of taking on too many patients, you will end up exhausted. Remember your priorities and the role that you want your job to play in your life. By chasing every dollar, your actions say that money wins out above your happiness, work-life balance, and even your health.

What About Practicing Part-Time?

Referring patients out to other dentists or reducing the treatments that you offer could be the first step to a more balanced, healthier career. If you are unsure about your next moves, but you want to reduce stress, try this first. If you still don't feel satisfied, consider other ways that you can "scale back" and reduce your hours at the office. Do you get joy out of being a dentist? If your answer is, "Yes, but..." it might be time to practice part-time.

You may come to the conclusion that dentistry provides you joy, but only when you have the time to treat a handful of patients without a lot of rush. Dentists may enjoy practicing in moderation, rather than devoting 40-50 hours a week and treating a revolving door of patients. Try finding an associate position that allows you to keep practicing but without the stress of a full-time non-stop commitment.

Do not shy away from researching part-time positions just because you do not want to take a pay cut. DSOs or individual dentists who need extra help may offer part-time positions that offer benefits, including:

- Guaranteed salary or commission
- 401(k) contributions
- CE allowance
- Flexible schedule

- Healthcare insurance

- Paid vacation days

Part-time hours could also give you the time that you need to explore other careers without completely walking away from your dentistry salary. Starting a business, freelancing, or selling real estate is not lucrative immediately, therefore keeping your day job might come in handy.

Completely Leaving

This chapter about partially leaving dentistry could feel like a waste of time. You have exhausted efforts to negotiate the terms of your position, and you know that even working part-time will fill you with dread. Entering dentistry, you felt hope and passion. Now, you wonder how you felt *anything* when thinking about teeth. You probably come to the conclusion that you've been sold on a lie; one that made promises of balanced work-lifestyle with nice cars and minimal debt. It's like buying into a game that is rigged from the start. The financial costs of your degree do not begin to cover the mental and emotional costs of tossing and turning over a workplace that doesn't fulfill you. You worked to earn a specific set of skills, but limitations from the employers you work for aren't allowing you to even *use* those skills to help others. Or you just found you really don't care about teeth and cavities.

Do not let yourself suffer in a job that doesn't bring you any joy or fulfillment. If you are feeling this way, it's probably time to leave the industry for good.

Signs It's Time to Leave Your Job

The decision to leave an esteemed industry like dentistry is not an easy one to make. As I addressed in Chapter 2, dentists often feel pressured to stay in their job because of the salary and status that comes from being a dentist. Friends, family, and colleagues may try to persuade you away from leaving. They may offer the same tips about negotiation or scaling back. I'm here to tell you that their advice may be helpful, but should not be the sole reason that you stay in a job that is killing you. If you are experiencing any of these feelings, it's in your best interest to move onto a new career.

You Have Reached All of the Milestones You Want to Reach

Ask yourself these three questions:

- Would you like to progress further in your field?

- Do you want to be in the shoes of people "higher up" within the next few years?

- What are you working toward when you go into the office every day?

Take money out of your answers. If your paycheck, or the hopes of a higher paycheck, is the only reason that you are driving to work every day, you may be missing out on other benefits that a job can bring you. (I'm not just talking about healthcare, either!) Think about the mental, physical, and emotional costs of your job. Is your paycheck covering all of these costs? Or is it time to stop "spending" your mental and emotional energy in a position with few rewards?

211

You have the ability to develop a passion for a new job position. When you decide to shift your goals and focus on a new career, you also provide yourself with the opportunity to set goals and reach milestones that you have not achieved. These achievements will not come without hard work and some stress, but you will have goals to work toward. Goals will give you a sense of direction and purpose. Practicing dentistry today with strictly monetary goals, or no goals at all fails to counteract the mental tolls of a stressful job position.

Stress from Work Affecting the Home

In Chapter 3, I addressed the physical toll of dentistry. Although the consequences of poor posture can be concerning, the consequences of little sleep are downright disturbing. When you bring the stress of a job home with you (and into bed with you,) you can put yourself at serious risk for numerous health conditions. By tossing and turning all night from stress, you are literally allowing a job to kill you. Do not let stress follow you home.

During my career as a full-time dentist, I rarely took vacation days. Most of my time was spent at work instead of at home. When I was away from the office, I was still "on call." Colleagues and referring dentists could reach me anytime. I never felt disconnected from work, even on those rare occasions when I did leave the state or the country.

■■

The connection to work got in the way of my connection to my family and friends.

■■

I brought stress everywhere I went, and that stress rubbed off on the people who were trying to include me in their life.

Have a conversation with your partner or your friends. Do you bring stress home from the office? Does stress from work affect your ability to communicate, relax, or fulfill your responsibilities at home? Work should be left at work. If the pressures of your job are routinely following you home, take a step back, and assess whether it's time to hit the "reset" button on your job.

You Wouldn't Recommend the Job to Your Friends or Children

If your friend was considering a career change, would you point them toward dental school? What would you tell your child if they said they wanted to be a dentist? Would you be happy sending your child off to dental school, knowing what you know now about student loans and the "costs" of a career in dentistry?

If the answer to these questions is "yes," think about *why* you would recommend dental school to your child. Among these reasons may be the benefits that keep you at your job. If the answer is "no," consider parting ways the profession. We sacrifice a lot for our children, but there is no reason to stay in a job that you would not recommend to your own child.

Deep Down, You Know That This Is the Right Thing to Do

When I am asked about my decision to step away from dentistry, I cite a number of reasons:

- I didn't feel that I was getting the respect I deserved from patients, despite excellent rapport and bed side manner.

- Insurance and DSOs, rather than dental expertise, were dictating what treatments each patient should receive.

- Malpractice suits are on the rise.

- I felt an increasing amount of back pain from long hours on my feet.

- The stress of performing a perfect treatment and getting perfect results was negatively affecting my mental health.

- The passion I had for dentistry when I began my career had gone away.

You do not have to cite one "perfect" reason for why you need to leave dentistry. A collection of small reasons still validates your choice to leave your current career or take a major step back. Do not let the opinions of someone who has not experienced a career in dentistry tell you that the mental, physical, or emotional toll of the career is minimal. They will inevitably exclaim, "I can't believe you went through all that extra schooling and took on all that debt just to quit!" Do not give these statements much weight. Your experiences are valid, and the choice to leave the career is yours, especially if it ultimately makes you happier.

If your "gut feeling" is telling you to leave your job, listen to it. Your body knows when something isn't right. Your body and mind do not want to be overwhelmed with stress. Listen to your body and take the steps to transition into a job that is less stressful, more fulfilling, and offers more chances for you to work toward something greater.

Ready to Leave Your Job? Get to Work

Securing a job as a dentist required years of hard work, education, and dedication. You didn't just tell people that you were going to become a dentist; you acted upon it. As you step into a new time in your life, you will need to find a career that gives you the same kind of hope and excitement that fueled you through dental school and beyond. You will need to take action, take risks, and be patient along the way. Transitioning into a new career may also take months or years. This journey begins with the decision that you are making as you read this book.

In the next chapter, I will share the story of how I scaled back and transformed my focus to a more engaging, fulfilling, and exciting career. My story may look similar to your story, but it won't be identical.

■■

The decision to leave a job is a personal decision.

■■

The next steps you take will depend on your interests, the passion you want to develop, and what you need to enjoy a fulfilling career *and* life.

Do not set off on this new journey alone. Once you have made the decision to leave your job or switch to part-time, tell people that you trust. A supportive group of friends, family members, or like-minded people should want to help you through this transition. Conversely, do not confine in those who will shame you or your decision. Make sure you tell people you trust about your intentions, plans, and feelings. Ask for help. This transition does not have to be kept secret. I could not have transitioned out of dentistry as successfully as I did without the help of my wife, friends, and colleagues. Most people who have made similar career changes will share the same sentiments.

Leaving dentistry may take a while to accomplish. You will need to create a plan and hold yourself accountable as you follow through with saving money, researching new careers, or applying for new positions. The support of friends and family can help you through this transition period. And remember, you are not the first dentist to step away from their career. You won't be the last, either.

Chapter 10:

Planning for a Change

Plan for what is difficult while it is easy. Do what is great while it is small.

— Sun Tzu

M y transition out of a full-time career in dentistry started a few years ago. I was working in corporate dentistry as a traveling periodontist going to multiple locations. I tried going into the office every day with a positive attitude but in fact, that proved to be challenging most of the time. Many of my colleagues had started to leave dentistry completely or shift to part time and I didn't understand why. When I first recognized this unhappiness within the profession, I internalized it and examined it. After a few years, I started to vocalize some concerns with dentistry here and there as I discussed my job with other providers. This was an enormous turning point in my career (and my life.)

I wasn't the only unhappy clinician, but I only discovered this when I started voicing my opinions. Other dentists expressed their grievances and why they were leaving the field, and I felt the support and validation that I had been silently seeking for months. Finally, I could talk to people who understood the severity of the tolls of being a dentist. Those who had left or scaled back were significantly happier and pursuing passions that fulfilled them. One of my friends from dental school actually sold his practice and decided he wanted to help young dentists become dental practice owners and build financial freedom. Another dentist I know who left dentistry started manufacturing reusable, clear face masks during the pandemic. I even talked to multiple dentists that left dentistry only to spend more time with their family. With this support, I decided to take things a step further and brainstorm ways to enjoy a more fulfilling career and life.

Maybe you have already expressed your frustrations with colleagues, friends, or family. Maybe you have kept these feelings to yourself out of fear or guilt. Do not repress these feelings any longer. I have seen many clinicians not only express their feelings but act on them. Some clinicians took other jobs, retired early, or even went back to school. Even before the COVID-19 pandemic, my colleagues were making these moves and setting themselves on a path toward a more fulfilling and satisfying career. Now, it's your turn. If you have decided that you need to leave your job, it's time to make some big moves.

Do not be mistaken. Big moves do not happen overnight. Each of these "big moves" consists of much smaller, incremental moves that you have to act upon every day. With the right mindset, some patience, and a clear direction, those big moves will turn into the best results you can imagine: a job (and life) that meets your top priorities and expectations.

These "big moves" include:

1. Saving enough money to leave your job (and not go back immediately)

2. Discover the path that is right for you

3. Make a time-bound plan with actionable items that will allow you to get the job you want

It's All About the Money: Saving Enough to Leave Your Job

Before I decided to step back from dentistry, I was in a "saving" mindset. I was not the dentist who opened a practice, and immediately went out to buy a Rolex. My frugality became a high priority when my child was born and I started paying for diapers. Saving up enough to work part-time was an easier transition for me than most.

Give yourself a few months to assess what you want to do. During that time, you can start to save money and prepare your family financially for your transition out of your job. Finding a new job may require some time without *any* job. If you do not properly save before this transition, you may find yourself returning to dentistry and accepting a lower-paying job out of desperation.

How to Save Up for a New Job

This financial security was a top priority during my transition out of clinical dentistry full-time. When I decided I needed to change careers, I had a stay-at-home wife and a young child that were relying on me for food, shelter, and other purchases. Saving my money was not always easy, but it was possible. Within six to nine months, I had the cushion I needed to comfortably walk away from my job if I chose to pursue a full-time career.

Financial experts recommend that you have around enough money to last you for six months after you quit your job.

■■■

If you have not taken the suggestion to assess your
current (or ideal) budget, do it now!

■■■

Carefully track how much money you are spending each
month. Track how much money is going to subscriptions,
savings, debt, and other recurring expenses. Understanding your
budget is key to searching for the right salary, paying off debt
faster, and having a cushion that will support you if you decide
to leave your job for good. Take advantage of resources like
www.biggerpockets.com or *www.whitecoatinvestor.com*, which
contains tons of helpful advice and many strategies towards
achieving financial goals.

Do not be discouraged if you need a few months (or even
years) to save this money. I had prioritized saving throughout
my career, and it *still* took me several months to put away my
ideal dollar amount. The more time you spend saving, the more
comfortable you will feel when you finally walk away from a
career that has been causing you physical and mental stress. I
saved for over nine months.

In addition to saving up to cover monthly expenses, I
also saved another set of money to cover any future investments
or business projects that would become a part of my new career.
You do not have to wait six months between quitting your own
job and finding a new job. You may begin earning income the
day after you quit the dental industry. Six months' worth of
living expenses in the bank simply provides a cushion for you to
explore new passions or look for another career. The more you
can put away toward a new business venture or investing, the
sooner you will be able to see money coming back to you.

220

Passive Income

Passive income is any money you earn through another source other than your employer. This could be anything from rental properties to stock dividends. Passive income opportunities may need some investment and a lot of development in the beginning. However, once these projects are off and running, these income avenues start to grow and are able to preserve themselves, bringing you a steady income with little effort from you. Creating an avenue for supplementary income can be a valuable source of funds for you while figuring out your next career move. Passive income can be just the thing to allow some cash flow after you leave clinical dentistry or otherwise experience some other financial hardship.

Take a look at these passive income ideas as you start planning for your career change:

1. Dividend Stocks

2. Peer to Peer Lending

3. Rental Properties

4. High Yield Savings Accounts And Money Market Funds

5. CD Ladders

6. Annuities

7. Invest Automatically In The Stock Market

8. Invest In A REIT

9. Refinance Your Mortgage

10. Pay Off Or Reduce Debt

11. Invest In A Business

12. Sell an eBook Online

13. Create a Course on Udemy

14. Selling Stock Photos

15. Licensing Music

16. Create an App

17. Affiliate Marketing

18. Network Marketing

19. Design T-Shirts

20. Sell Digital Files on Etsy

21. List Your Place On Airbnb

22. Car Wash

23. Rent Out Your Car

24. Vending Machines

25. Storage Rentals

26. Laundromat

27. Cashback Rewards Cards

28. Cashback Sites

29. Get Paid To Have An App On Your Phone

30. Save Up To 30% On Your Electric Bill

Tips for Saving

Once you have a number in mind (and a set number of months for you to save,) it's time to get frugal.

Assess your interest. It is much easier to save money when you do not have to pay off any debt. Financial experts recommend that you start with the debt that has the highest interest rates. In previous chapters, I have addressed refinancing or choosing an income-based repayment plan. If you have not already considered these strategies, you might want to revisit them. Consolidating your debt may also be a helpful strategy as you get serious about saving (and your budget overall.) As you start to slash monthly spending, take a portion of what you have saved, and pay off your debt faster.

Ask for a raise. Even if you do not plan to stay at your job for more than a year or two, ask for a raise. The more money you collect each month (without working extra hours,) the more you can save. Do not let your plans to leave the dental industry hold you back from asking for the money that you deserve.

Keep track of *every* purchase. Budgeting apps make it easy to assess how much you are spending each month, but many people believe they make it *too* easy. If you want to motivate yourself to stop spending, start physically writing down *each purchase that you make.* Keep a spreadsheet or a journal. Every time you make a purchase or see a recurring expense pop up on your bank statement, write it down. Not only will you be less motivated to make the purchase in the first place, but you will also physically see what is eating away at your budget each month.

Minimize subscriptions. It's easy to subscribe to a streaming platform, fitness center, or other subscription services. Do not let these purchases eat away at your savings - especially if you are not using them. Downgrading my TV plan and minimizing other subscriptions was crucial to helping me save some extra cash each month. If you see a recurring expense that is not necessary, cancel it immediately. Do not wait for the next billing cycle, because you will probably forget. Drop everything you can live without and cancel those unnecessary subscriptions.

Plan your expenses - to the week.
Break your spending down to each individual purchase. How much are you spending on groceries this week? On dining out? Vet bills? That gym membership that you aren't using? How much are you going to put into a savings account? (If you don't have a savings account, open one up. The reward of transferring money into a savings account will motivate you further.) The more control you have over your expenses, the easier it will be to curb unnecessary spending.

Live like a dental student. You have lived with minimal expenses before (or fewer expenses than you do now.) Get back into the mindset that you had in dental school. Remember that your priorities lie in saving up for a more lucrative future, not spending what you have in the moment.

Once again, the right mindset can help you reach your goals faster. Get into the habit of assessing your spending and opting out of more expensive options. Keep your end goal in mind - and the sweet feeling of choosing a career that makes *you* happy.

Assess Your Situation

Saving an appropriate amount of money to quit your job may take months. Use this time to explore alternative careers. If you quit your job *before* forming a back-up plan, you'll blow through your savings before you are able to earn a steady income. Your back-up plan will also give you an insight on whether you can quit your job completely *or* switch to part-time.

After I decided to step away from clinical dentistry full-time, I enlisted the help of friends, colleagues, and my wife. We assessed my current priorities in life. Fellow dentists and I shared our struggles with our job positions and brainstormed ideas for projects outside of the office. We swapped career assessments and other tools that pointed us in a direction toward a dream career.

I have mentioned a few of these resources in previous chapters. Different assessments will prove to be more or less helpful, depending on how much direction you need and where you might want to go.

These assessments told me a few things:

- I wanted to explore entrepreneurship and owning my own business

- A flexible schedule (and the opportunity to spend more time with my family) is a top priority for me

- I would make sacrifices and undergo some levels of stress to make a decent income

- Small amounts of stress are manageable if they lead me to fulfilling projects and achievements

There is an infinite number of jobs that I could take. By taking career assessments, I narrowed down my options to a handful of careers or business ventures. All of these choices fit my priorities: I could enjoy time with my family by working flexible hours and making a decent income. But some choices required more time, education, and attention than others.

Weighing the Pros and Cons

In addition to taking personality assessments, my colleagues and I shared ideas about where to go next. We all had different priorities and goals for our career. Some people wanted to stay in the world of dentistry and found themselves weighing the options that I shared in Chapter 8. Others prioritized going back to school. Even though we all *started* in similar positions, the handful of jobs that seemed most appropriate for us varied from person to person.

A handful of jobs is not a solid backup plan, but it's a start. In order to narrow down my choices for a post-dentistry career, I made a "pros and cons" list. On separate sheets of paper, I wrote down a handful of jobs that fit my priorities and listed all of the benefits and the drawbacks. Among my choices were entering into investment realty, different entrepreneurial ventures, and one or two "9 to 5" positions that allowed me to work remotely. I had some clear favorites before writing my lists but wanted to keep an open mind. The choice that I *wanted* to pursue may not have been the most practical, and a "pros and cons" list would physically show that to me.

You have probably made a "pros and cons" list before. This form of decision-making is free and accessible, but *preparation* is what makes it effective. Anyone can make a "pros and cons" list for a handful of jobs, but this list is as far as many people go. Take things one step further by truly looking at each "pro" and "con." In order to see how they fit into your life, you

225

will need to have already assessed your priorities and figured out the salary you need to live comfortably. If you have not already made a list of your priorities and truly thought about what is important in your career and your life, you have some work to do.

One of the potential careers on my list was owning a dental career coaching and consulting business. For me, calling the shots and starting the business was a "pro." Other dentists who might feel burnt out or just unfulfilled by running their own practice may see entrepreneurship as a "con." A job's features and benefits could be a "pro" or "con" depending on the individual writing the list. Another "pro" of starting this business was the opportunity for growth. I was starting with nothing. I liked the idea of having smaller goals grow into larger ones. Again, this could be a drawback for someone who wants to minimize stress.

■■■

Be realistic with each potential job that interests you.

■■■

Do not hesitate to list "cons," even if your heart is telling you to take that job. I really wanted to start my own coaching business, but knew that six-figure paychecks would not roll in immediately. Simply neglecting this drawback could have set me up for financial failure. If I wanted to make the income that could support me, my wife, and my child, I would need another gig. One "con" is not a reason to abandon your dreams of a different job. You should *address* said "con" as you move forward, but do not let it stop you from making the career change you need and deserve.

Finding additional sources of income were necessary, so I combined a few potential jobs that also allowed me to have a flexible schedule while developing my passions and earning

Income. After carefully calculating my options, I realized that practicing as a clinician two days a week would be the "missing piece" to the puzzle of my career. Dentistry could not consume my life anymore. I could practice as a hobby while focusing more of my time and energy on alternative careers. As I grew my career coaching business, the money I earned from dentistry would be less of a cushion and more of a bonus. If I wanted to walk away altogether, I could. (I would probably create another "pros and cons" list first, just in case!)

Although the initial brainstorm should be done amongst colleagues and friends, consider writing your "pros and cons" list by yourself. Again, a "pro" for you might be a "con" for someone else. Keep your list of priorities nearby. Is each potential job allowing you to focus on what really matters to you? Could the job elevate one aspect of your life, while pushing another aspect into the shadows? Consider all of your priorities and everything we have discussed in this book (the mental, physical, and emotional toll a job can take on you) as you are writing your list.

A "pros and cons" list can be a physical representation of how a job will make you feel once you pursue it. Be thorough, and spend as much time thinking about every potential job on your list. You'll see the pros pile up on some jobs, and the cons pile up on the others. If two jobs are vying for your top choice, consider the *weight* of each pro and con on your list. The more that you compare a handful of jobs, the more obvious the choice will become.

Give It A Try

You know firsthand that the career that you envision as a student may not be the career that you have experienced as an adult. College courses don't tell you how to deal with finicky patients or handle the guilt that comes with being everyone's worst fear. Before you dive into a new career, dip your toes into the water. Give yourself the freedom to experience a job without committing to it. If you come to find that your new venture isn't as enjoyable as you imagined, you will save yourself the time and money of pivoting only to pivot a few months later.

This type of "research" will require that you find people who are already working in this field. Set up Zoom calls or coffee dates and ask about the day-to-day responsibilities of the job. Ask about the most stressful things that people experience. Shadow or intern with someone for a day to see what *you* will be doing day in and day out. Take up some work on the side and see how it feels to try something new.

A mentorship can be your connection to all of these opportunities. Seek out someone who has the time and passion to mentor you. They can help you determine whether a job is right for you and create the best strategies for pivoting. Mentorships are extremely valuable.

■■

Do not underestimate what a good mentor can do to help you move forward in your new career.

■■

Make a Plan

You do not have to take assessments, brainstorm jobs, and create "pros and cons" lists all in one night. Take your time choosing which direction you want to go after you have quit your job. Your first choice may quickly turn out to be the wrong choice - that's why saving for at least six months' worth of income is so important before you walk away from your job. Be patient.

Once you have made your choice, you're not done preparing. Work with your mentor and make a plan before you quit. You'll quickly need to put it in action. This plan should consist of a timeline and a list of tasks that will need to be completed before you start applying for jobs or opening your own business. As you save and wait for the perfect time to walk away, make sure you check off every one of these tasks. Again, these might not be overnight projects. Use this transition period as a time to explore your contributions as an employee, recognize your skills, and communicate your value to people who may want to employ you or work with you in the future.

Top tasks that should be in your plan include:

- Updating your resume
- Evaluating your talents
- Scheduling interview prep
- Learning additional skills
- Assess your realistic and ideal salary
- Networking and discussing your plan to others

Update Your Resume (Not Your CV)

If you are opening up your own practice, you don't need to show your resume to anyone. You're the boss. DSOs and established private dental practices may seek you out based on your experience, rapport, and location. Dentists who are looking for a clinical career within an established organization may create a *curriculum vitae* (CV) to show to potential employers. CVs usually contain:

- Education and CE information

229

- List of professional licenses (and when they were updated)
- Career goals or a personal statement
- List of appearances in medical journals or publications
- Residency information
- Practice ownership or employment history
- Professional membership or community service history

CVs are common amongst dentists and other healthcare professionals, but not the document of choice among other employers. Unless you are going into academia or law, you should convert your CV into a resume. Resumes, rather than CVs, are usually requested by employers in sales, business, real estate, and most other industries. If you submit a CV to a non-clinical employer, you are quickly telling them that you're new to the job hunt.

Resumes and CVs contain similar information, including a list of degrees and a history of professional experience. The formatting for resumes and CVs differs slightly. Resumes are typically one page, while CVs may contain multiple pages with a list of publications and other academic achievements. If you are pivoting toward a career in academia (as mentioned in Chapter 8,) keep your CV. Otherwise, consult a career coach on how to convert your CV into a resume. Take a quick look below to see the differences between a resume and a CV.

Resume	CV
Showcases competence: work history and accomplishments, etc.	Showcases credentials: certifications, research, affiliations, etc.
Summary of skills and experience relevant to the position	Comprehensive history of life's work and education
Used for practically any job	Used for academic, scientific, and medial jobs

Evaluate Your Skills – And the Skills Employers Want to See

Job seekers may have two or three versions of their resume, each slightly tweaked for different companies or job positions. A resume tailored for work at a nonprofit, for example, may highlight different experiences than a resume tailored for work at a Fortune 500 company. If you are sending in a resume for a position that requires knowledge of the dental industry, you might highlight your education and license renewals. As you are building different versions of your resume, you will need to understand what you can bring to each potential job.

Look at what *you* can bring to the table and what employers *want* you to bring to the table. If you are transitioning out of dentistry into a career outside of healthcare, you may need to think outside the box. Yes, you may be a dentist and you may have spent four years developing the ability to perform a root canal or a cavity prep. Employers outside of dentistry don't need you to put those skills on your resume. Think about the skills you developed while working at your practice, making decisions,

231

or solving problems. Do you have a knack for fostering communication or creating action-based solutions? Are you organized? Disciplined? What kind of leadership style do you prefer to use?

These are the skills that employers across different industries want to know when they look at your application.

■■■

A thorough evaluation of your skills can help you craft the perfect resume.

■■■

Although, you need to do more than just write "good with people," or "learns fast" under your "skills." Employers want *proof* that you are good with people or that you learn fast. They want to see how your skills translate into tangible results. When they see the results you have brought to other employers, they will see the value that you can bring to *them*. (The higher they value you, the more they will offer.)

Make a list of your achievements at work. What reviews did patients leave about their experience with you? If your employer could name three skills that you bring to the office, what would they say? Have you received any awards or recognitions based on particular skills? Were up able to implement changes that increased patients or treatment acceptance? Keep these skills in mind as you look for jobs and create your resume.

Are your skills and traits important? Check job listings. Browse through job descriptions and requirements for jobs that you want to hold. (No need to apply yet. Just do some research.) What skills continue to make an appearance on job listings? What do employers want to see? These skills could range from "ability to work on a team" to "knack for catching small mistakes." Utilize these job listings as you list your skills and prior responsibilities on your resume.

Schedule Some Interview Prep

Understanding your skills is the first step in showing an employer that you have skills. Adding them to your resume is another step. But expert career coaches suggest that the most important thing you can do with your skills is to *demonstrate* them in an interview. Interviews can be terrifying. If you want to get better at interviewing for your dream job, you've got to practice.

Career coaches can give you feedback on how you conduct yourself in an interview. Do you know who can also give you feedback? Employers. Even if you are not completely ready to apply for jobs and leave your current one, apply anyway. Go for an interview, even if you do not want the job. Employers expect to be asked for feedback from potential candidates and may give you the advice you need to score your dream job in two or three month's time.

Start Networking

I would not have been as motivated to leave my job if it weren't from the support, ideas, and resources provided by my colleagues. These were friends that had similar feeling about the state of dentistry and who were contemplating leaving or had already left.

A strong network of professionals is key to successfully leaving your job and creating a solid plan to enjoy a new venture.

∎∎

If you are not connected with professionals in the dental industry (or the industry that you want to enter) it's time to start networking.

Networking opportunities are everywhere. Young kids have even turned to *dating* apps to make professional connections. (Bumble Bizz separates people who use the app for dates and those who want to network.) Search for events, both online and in-person, that bring professionals together. Coworking spaces, cultural hubs, and alumni centers are great places to start looking for events. Keep an eye out for these events, or reach out to people in your community for recommendations. Use social media forums or groups to reach out to others and learn more about a particular industry.

Friends, family, and colleagues can give you advice on how to have a great interview. They can also look over your resume, send you job opportunities, and refer you to professionals in the field that you want to enter. They won't do any of these things, however, if you don't let them know that you are exploring other careers.

Chapter 6 addresses how difficult this can be for dentists. Dentists are in an esteemed position, with a typically high salary. Friends and family outside of the dentistry world may be confused as to why a dentist would want to leave their job and explore a potentially less lucrative career. Do not let this type of skepticism hold you back from potentially gaining contacts, referrals, and other connections that can lead you in the right direction.

The best way to "defend" against skeptics is to have a solid plan in place. If you know your budget and the job that will replace your current one, you will have all the answers to questions you may receive. Skeptics cannot poke too many holes in a plan that is solid. The more you have planned, the more people in your circle will trust you and help you through your journey. Preparing for your pivot is crucial to making it happen.

Evaluate Your Mindset

A solid plan and preparation will set you up for a smooth transition, but all of this will crumble if you do not have the right mindset. Your mindset is the foundation for anything you want to build.

■■■

If your mindset is strong, you can brush off anything that threatens your happiness or progress as you make a successful career change.

■■■

You will face threats along the way. Never mind the doubts or pressure from family and friends. Throughout this process, *you* will likely face your own doubts and fears. You will question yourself, and consider crawling back to a "safe" career that has at least produced a paycheck in the past. Do not let these questions or fears overcome you. You have made it this far. I do not doubt that you have already faced doubts or voices in your head telling you that you will be judged harshly by other people. These doubts have not held you back in the past. Do not let them hold you back now.

235

Affirmations, stress reduction, and support from others can help to build a strong foundation and mindset moving forward. Remind yourself that you have the right to change careers. People grow and pursue new interests and ways of earning money. You are growing and changing, too. Repeat this idea to yourself *every day* to solidify this mindset. As you strengthen the ideas that you deserve this career change, you will be able to stay disciplined and do the work necessary to successfully shift to the career of your dreams.

ACTIVITY: Here is a short quiz to help you determine your current satisfaction level in dentistry. Circle the answers that most closely reflect the way you feel and follow the directions after answering to see your results.

1. I enjoy performing dental procedures:

   a. Strongly Agree
   b. Agree
   c. Undecided
   d. Disagree
   e. Strongly Disagree

2. I like working with patients:

   a. Strongly Agree
   b. Agree
   c. Undecided
   d. Disagree
   e. Strongly Disagree

3. I make the money that I deserve:

   a. Strongly Agree
   b. Agree
   c. Undecided
   d. Disagree
   e. Strongly Disagree

4. I am physically capable of working in dentistry for a long time:

   a. Strongly Agree
   b. Agree
   c. Undecided
   d. Disagree
   e. Strongly Disagree

5. I look forward to coming into the office each day:

   a. Strongly Agree
   b. Agree
   c. Undecided
   d. Disagree
   e. Strongly Disagree

6. I have always wanted to be a dentist:

   a. Strongly Agree
   b. Agree
   c. Undecided
   d. Disagree
   e. Strongly Disagree

7. I am passionate about oral healthcare:

   a. Strongly Agree
   b. Agree
   c. Undecided
   d. Disagree
   e. Strongly Disagree

8. I have excellent staff and assistants:

   a. Strongly Agree
   b. Agree
   c. Undecided
   d. Disagree
   e. Strongly Disagree

9. I have a flexible schedule that allows me to not feel overworked:

   a. Strongly Agree
   b. Agree
   c. Undecided
   d. Disagree
   e. Strongly Disagree

10. I could be happy with dentistry if I just changed employers:

    a. Strongly Agree
    b. Agree
    c. Undecided
    d. Disagree
    e. Strongly Disagree

11. I am comfortable with the stability of my job:

    a. Strongly Agree
    b. Agree
    c. Undecided
    d. Disagree
    e. Strongly Disagree

12. My family and friends would not be supportive if I left dentistry:

    a. Strongly Agree
    b. Agree
    c. Undecided
    d. Disagree
    e. Strongly Disagree

Add up the number of answer choices selected and multiply by the number given. Then add the numbers in the right-hand column for a grand total.

$$a = \underline{\hspace{1cm}} \times 1 = \underline{\hspace{1cm}}$$
$$b = \underline{\hspace{1cm}} \times 2 = \underline{\hspace{1cm}}$$
$$c = \underline{\hspace{1cm}} \times 3 = \underline{\hspace{1cm}}$$
$$d = \underline{\hspace{1cm}} \times 4 = \underline{\hspace{1cm}}$$
$$e = \underline{\hspace{1cm}} \times 5 = \underline{\hspace{1cm}}$$

_____ **TOTAL**

0-20: Congratulations! You probably have it pretty good and should stay in dentistry! Why did you buy this book?!

21-40: It's time to modify your situation so that you can leave dentistry partly or stay in dentistry but under some new terms and conditions.

41-60: Did you even need this quiz to tell you that being a dentist isn't all it's cracked up to be for you? Leaving dentistry completely should be your new goal. Why waste another minute doing something that doesn't make you happy? Time to hang up your explorer.

Ready, Set, Go!

Expect people to question your departure away from dentistry, but do not take their skepticism personally. For years, people have been told that dentistry is the nicest gig around. The people who question your choice to leave may not understand that "sweet" is not the best word to describe dentistry. And ultimately, the choice is yours. Your priorities may not line up with a close friend or a family member. The role you want your job to play in your life may differ from the role your partner or colleague wants a career to play in their life. You are the only one that can make a list of your priorities *and* take the steps to meet them. Colleagues, family members, and supportive individuals will help to hold you accountable and support you along this process.

Conclusion

Some tortures are physical
And some are mental,
But the one that is both
Is dental.

— **Ogden Nash**

This book provides a *lot* of information, resources, and strategies that can help you assess your career goals. Do not be overwhelmed. I do not include any due dates in this book for a reason. The time you need to make a list of your priorities, pursue the career of your dreams, and live a satisfying life depends on where you are today. My transformation began three years ago. If I had never questioned my career or dentistry's role in my life, my pivot would have never happened at all.

Your journey starts with just one question:

Do you still *enjoy* clinical dentistry?

If you took the time to read this book, you *probably* don't enjoy everything about your career in clinical dentistry. But many people can get caught up in thinking that the grass is greener on the other side. All jobs come with some amount of stress. Pinpoint what exactly stresses *you* out about your job in order to see the "grass" where you're standing. If you do enjoy dentistry, but don't enjoy certain things that you can change by switching jobs or asking for a raise, you might not need to take a huge leap into a new field.

Do you not like your front desk staff or your dental assistants? Rather than save up money to step away from dentistry entirely, you may just need to spend some time searching for a position within another DSO. Do you still get fired up talking about oral health, but tense up at the thought of tough patients and insurance companies? Consider the pros and cons of switching to a career in academia, where you can share your love of dentistry with students who are developing their own passion. Does the thought of working at *any* clinic, or continuing your education in the world of dentistry fill you with dread? You might need to take a step back and figure out what brings you joy in life.

■■■

Once you have considered what you want, take a break and stop there.

■■■

Deciding what you want out of your career is a different process than building the strategies to get you there. Once you have unapologetically and confidently declared (to yourself or others) what you want out your career, celebrate. Throughout this book, I have discussed the guilt and shame that many dentists feel about wanting to transition out of dentistry. Understanding and speaking to what you want, especially if it involves a major career change, is a big step to take. Celebrate. Take your time before you develop a time-bound and structured plan to pivot. We are starting to transition out of a time where *everything* was uncertain. Take advantage of this global shake-up and strategically, intentionally choose your next moves.

Now Is the Best Time to Make a Change

In 2020, the COVID-19 pandemic flipped the world upside down. Over 40 million Americans lost their jobs. The ones who were lucky enough to *keep* their non-essential jobs were sent home for weeks, months, or indefinitely. Zoom calls replaced morning meetings. "Slack" took on a whole new meaning. Professionals in healthcare became overwhelmed with work *or* twiddled their thumbs, waiting for the day that they could reopen their practice.

Dentists found themselves faced with a new opportunity: the opportunity to bow out gracefully from their job without being questioned. Pre-COVID, dentists would face scrutiny or guilt for exiting a career that came with high esteem and a six-figure salary. This guilt wasn't just a feeling - it felt like a trap for millennials and dentists who felt fooled by the "Golden Age of Dentistry." Over the years, dentistry has become a trap with increasing mental, physical, and emotional pressures. After reading this book, I hope that you can see that dentistry isn't a trap, but merely one career path for people who feel passionate about oral health and helping others. If you have lost this passion, or feel weighed down by the stress of your career, you have other options.

This is not an easy thing to see in our society. The history of the 9-5 shows that employment terms and demands stem from national guidelines. Trends in loyalty and on-the-job pressure have not been going in a direction that benefits the employee.

242

Not only do patients feel as though they can demand more from their healthcare professionals, but people at the top also set precedents that include 40+ hour workweeks, staying "on-call" at all hours, and skipping the few vacation days allotted to employees. As a country, the average worker puts in more hours than workers in similarly developed countries. Dentists face higher pressures, and accept these higher pressures in exchange for the high rewards they are promised.

High rewards also come with the illusion of low turnover. Young adults may not be pressured to enter dental school, but are simply drawn in by the benefits of holding such an esteemed career. The promises given to students in dental school about the life of a dentist remain unfulfilled: freedom from the shackles of a traditional 9-5, financial independence, and the ability to serve a higher purpose. Dental students, seduced by these promises, willingly sign up for hundreds of thousands of dollars in student loan debt. At the time, these loans appear to be a small bump in the road. How hard could it be to pay back six figures when you're making six figures?

The "costs" of being a dentist, unfortunately, include more than just $300,000 in student loans. They include the pressure of perfecting each and every treatment. They include the literal costs of chiropractors, surgeons, and other treatments for physical ailments that come from standing all day. A six-figure salary, especially one that has remained stagnant since the Great Recession of 2008, will certainly not be able to cover the medical costs that come with the effects of chronic stress.

The costs of working for a DSO or running a private practice pile up faster and faster. The pressure to avoid malpractice suits and provide exceptional treatment and services day in and day out becomes a burden that is too heavy to carry.

Dentists often fail to acknowledge the effects of
carrying so much weight on their shoulders.

After all, their jobs are depicted as "perfect" and
"fulfilling" by specialists with high Instagram and Facebook
followers.

Everyone is searching for the perfect job. Everyone is
searching for the perfect work-life balance. This search is what
brought most people into dental school in the first place. Now,
dentistry is far from the "ideal" job. Programmers, tech whizzes,
and affiliate marketers now have the spotlight. Pre-COVID, they
were the few that could easily find a remote job, pack their bags,
and head to Thailand for a life of low expenses, high pay, and
location independence. One could only scroll through their
social media feed and dream about the possibility of working
from their computer on a beach or cafe 1,000 miles away.

The COVID-19 pandemic has forced a lot of companies
to show their employees that working from their computers *is*
possible. The world still needs to adjust to a constantly changing
"new normal," but more companies are allowing employees to
work from home indefinitely. Jobs that offer location
independence are easier to find than ever. An employee's value
is more likely to be defined by results, rather than physical
presence in a cubicle. Maybe COVID-19 was the shake-up that
business owners, employees, and even dentists needed to break
free from the more traditional working schedule. The future of
the "9 to 5" may not be bound to time at all.

What's Next?

What does *your* future look like? When you picture your "office" in one, five, or ten years, where do you go? When you retire for the night (or retire indefinitely,) how do you imagine reflecting on your career? Instead of reflecting on the accomplishments within your job, maybe you are more inclined to dream about what happens *outside* of work. How will your job shape the way that you are able to take care of your family, see the world, and truly experience the things you want out of life?

When you are young, you are expected to have the answers to these questions. During this time, you are expected to make the largest purchase of your life so that you can earn money in four years. When you chose dentistry or another career, you might not have *had* those answers. You may not even have them now. As you go through different experiences and try new things, you are likely to adjust or change the way that you view your career, work-life balance, and the ways that you want to show up for your family, community, and the world. COVID-19 shook up the way that Americans viewed the 9-5 workweek and how to maintain a healthy work-life balance. Use this time to not only adjust to your "new normal," but to figure out what that new normal looks like *for you.*

■■■

Do not rush into finding a new job.

■■■

After spending at least four years in dental school, you deserve to take some time to truly explore your options and find a career that suits you. You have options for staying in the dental field and using your degree *while working remotely* or fulfilling your passion. If you want to abandon any obligation to look into a patient's mouth, you have that option, too.

ACTIVITY: Career coach, Foram Sheth, shares seven questions you should ask yourself before you quit your job. Take a look and see if you can answer these questions:

1. What would it take for me to be happy at my current job/field?
2. Am I running away from something or toward something?
3. What problems do I expect by quitting my job to solve?
4. Can I defend my choice to leave even if others disagree?
5. Can I financially afford to quit?
6. What's my plan for day one after quitting?

Three years ago, I wasn't sure what the future had in store for me. All I knew was that I was tired of walking on eggshells around anxious patients and compromising my expertise so someone could increase their bottom line. Transitioning out of a full-time career in dentistry was daunting. How would I pay the bills? How could I avoid going *back* to a "9 to 5" with an organization that didn't have my best interests in mind? I didn't have the answers immediately. Neither will you. Three years later, I am still exploring new opportunities and building a career that is both lucrative *and* fulfilling. Dentistry is still a part of my life. Instead of hating every day that I step into the office, I have regained a love for the practice. Dentistry is now a fulfilling hobby. It's a way to connect with people in my community. Most importantly, it has inspired me to create my current venture: career coaching. In the past three years, I have been able to do all of these things and take back control over my schedule, finances, and work-life balance. Now, I want to do the same for you.

Checklist to a Successful Career Change

ACTIVITY: Review this checklist I've created for assessing your interests, exploring options, evaluating alternative career paths, and making the move out of dentistry and into a new career:

— **Assess your current job satisfaction.** Ask yourself if you are happy in the position you currently hold and in what areas would you like to see change.

— **Take inventory.** Determine what skills, values, and interests contributed to your success as a dentist and how they can apply to various roles you might be interested in. This is also an opportunity to assess your strengths and weaknesses.

— **Decide if you want to change industries.** Determine if staying in dentistry (clinical or non-clinical) is a possibility, or if leaving dentistry is ultimately what would make you happy.

— **Save.** Start saving every dime you can so you can live comfortably during the transition. This is also an opportunity to save for prospective investments you want to make during this time. It is advised that you may need to save for 9 months (or even longer) to have enough cushion depending on your lifestyle and circumstances.

— **Brainstorm careers.** Discuss potential career options that may interest you with friends and family. Do you want to work as an employee or start your own business as an entrepreneur?

— **Explore potential job matches.** Search online classifieds or job listings to see if the career you want is in demand.

— **Pick a career.** Select the career or job that most aligns with your goals and passions

— **Research.** Find out if any certifications, pre-requisites, or other qualifications are necessary for the career you want.

— **Create an action plan.** Set a timeline with actionable tasks to complete. Decide if and when you want to switch to part-time dentistry while you search for jobs. You might determine when the ideal time is for a change.

— **Rebrand yourself.** Update your resume to showcase non-dental skills that may interest employers.

— **Start networking.** Talk with others who have been your position or have the career you desire. This is a great opportunity to find a mentor that will assist you on your journey.

— **Look for hands-on opportunities.** Try finding workshops or apprenticeships in the field you want to pursue. Any experience can be a good experience.

— **Consider educational resources.** Think about if you should go back to school or at a minimum sign up for courses that will equip you with the training you need for your new career.

— **Develop new skills.** Acquire easy to learn skills that will advance your skill set in the field you desire to pursue.

— **Track your progress.** Seeing what tasks have been completed and what areas still need work is a great way to hold yourself accountable in reaching your goal of changing careers. How many applications have you submitted? How many interviews have you had?

After completing all these steps and still no luck, just rinse and repeat. Remember, switching careers and not for the faint and requires hard work and determination. Everyone's situation is different so feel free to modify these steps to your liking. You are in control of your destiny. As long as you have a plan, you are headed in the right direction!

Final Thoughts

I hope this book was able to give you enough information to adjust your thinking and look to the future with excitement. The infinite possibilities ahead are a breath of fresh air compared to the "trap" of dentistry. Exploring other careers and opportunities may feel like seeing the light for the first time in years. Embrace it. Take every moment to freely develop your passions and find out what priorities you want to focus on in the next few years.

For some, this book may have made you realize that leaving dentistry isn't realistic nor something you truly want. You may have come to the conclusion that the good parts about being a dentist outweigh the bad. You may have figured out that starting over is not something you have the desire or energy to undertake. If that is the case, then you should feel resolve in knowing that you are in the right career for you at this particular moment in your life. That is not to say, that things cannot change, but it's what works for now. If you have chosen to stay in dentistry, then I hope this book has motivated you to take action in creating a positive and enjoyable work environment that you deserve. Restructure your situation to where you dread the weekends and can't wait for Monday to come!

Put yourself at the center of this journey, but do not set off on it alone. The catalyst for leaving dentistry has also been the most rewarding part of my journey: my family. Reconnecting with my family and connecting with others has been my main source of motivation and inspiration over the past three years. By stepping back from my career, I was able to step up into my role as a husband and a father. There is still pressure that comes with these responsibilities, but the rewards are greater than anything that I could have ever imagined.

Reach out to the people who you care about most. Let them be the motivation that you need to leave your dental career. In two, three, five, or ten years, you will realize that leaving dentistry might have been the best thing that you've ever done. Whether you are still in dental school or have been practicing for decades, it's never too late to make career change.

Whatever your decision, it's important that you understand some very important things about yourself before you begin your new journey. You are not alone. There are hundreds who feel the same and welcome solidarity. You are extremely smart and capable, which is evident from your educational and work experience. You deserve to live the life you want to live, with the people you love, doing the thing you feel most passionate about. You are appreciative of all the things dentistry has bestowed upon you, but change is necessary. You are strong and motivated to find solutions to your situation that will ultimately work in your favor. Your dream career will become a reality. Being a dentist does not define you or control you. You control your destiny and you control if and when you want to leave the profession. You are the master of your destiny and all is possible when you commit to change. You are more than a dentist and soon everyone will know!

NOTES:

NOTES:

Printed in Great Britain
by Amazon

40603595R00145